This publication is intended to provide educational information for the reader on the covered subjects. It is not intended to take the place of personalized medical counseling, diagnosis, and treatment from a trained healthcare professional.

ISBN 978-1-7382732-7-0 (Hardcover)

ISBN 978-1-7382732-8-7 (Paperback)

ISBN 978-1-7382732-9-4 (eBook)

Printed and bound in USA

Published by Loons Press

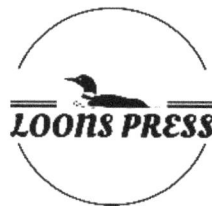

LOONS PRESS

TABLE OF CONTENTS

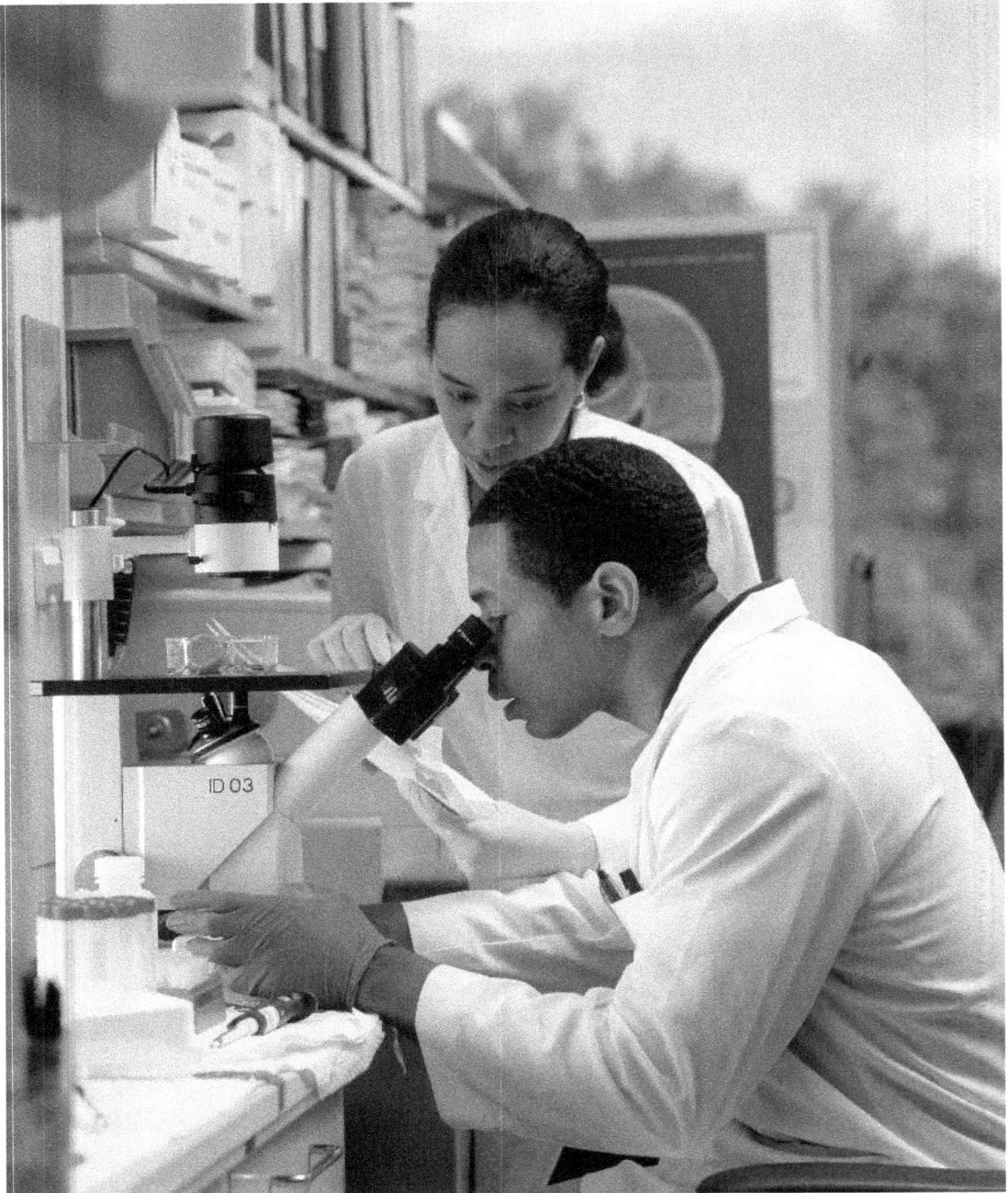

Chapter 1: Understanding Cancer

What is Cancer?

Cancer is a complex and devastating disease that affects millions of people worldwide. It is important for everybody to have a basic understanding of what cancer is, how it develops, and why early detection is crucial in improving outcomes. This subchapter aims to provide an overview of cancer, its causes, and the importance of being proactive in recognizing signs and symptoms sooner.

Cancer is a term used to describe a group of diseases characterized by the uncontrolled growth and spread of abnormal cells in the body. These abnormal cells, known as cancer cells, can invade and destroy nearby tissues and organs. If left untreated or undetected, cancer can metastasize, spreading to other parts of the body through the blood or lymphatic system.

The causes of cancer are multifactorial and can vary depending on the type of cancer. While some cancers may be hereditary, others are linked to lifestyle factors such as smoking, poor diet, lack of physical activity, exposure to certain chemicals or radiation, and infections. It is crucial to understand that not all cancers can be prevented, but adopting a healthy lifestyle and avoiding known risk factors can significantly reduce the chances of developing the disease.

Early detection of cancer plays a vital role in improving treatment outcomes and survival rates. Recognizing the signs and symptoms of cancer can lead to an earlier diagnosis, allowing for more effective treatment options. Common signs of cancer can include unexplained weight loss, persistent fatigue, changes in the skin, lumps or swelling, changes in bowel or bladder habits, persistent cough, and difficulty swallowing, among others. It is important to note that these symptoms can also be caused by non-cancerous conditions, but it is always better to be safe and consult a healthcare professional if any persistent or unexplained symptoms arise.

By being proactive and aware of the signs and symptoms of cancer, individuals can take control of their health and seek medical attention at the earliest indication of a problem. Regular screenings and check-ups are also essential, as they can help detect cancer in its early stages, often before symptoms manifest. Remember, knowledge is power, and being well-informed about cancer can empower individuals to take charge of their health, make informed decisions, and potentially save lives.

In conclusion, cancer is a complex and devastating disease that affects millions of people worldwide. By understanding what cancer is, its causes, and the importance of early detection, individuals can become proactive in recognizing signs and symptoms sooner. It is crucial for everybody to be aware of the common signs of cancer and to seek medical attention promptly if any concerning symptoms arise. Empower yourself and those around you with knowledge about cancer, as early detection can make a significant difference in treatment outcomes and overall survival rates.

Common Types of Cancer

Cancer is a widespread and complex disease that affects millions of people worldwide. It can strike anyone, regardless of age, gender, or lifestyle, making it crucial for everyone to be aware of the common types of cancer. Understanding these types can empower individuals to detect early signs and symptoms, leading to earlier diagnosis and potentially better treatment outcomes. This subchapter aims to provide a comprehensive overview of the most prevalent types of cancer and their associated signs.

Breast cancer is one of the most well-known types of cancer and affects both men and women. It usually manifests as a lump or thickening in the breast tissue, but other symptoms, such as nipple discharge or changes in breast shape, may also indicate its presence. Regular breast self-examinations and mammograms are essential for early detection.

Lung cancer is primarily caused by smoking, but non-smokers can also develop this disease. Persistent cough, chest pain, and shortness of breath are common symptoms. Early detection is crucial for successful treatment, as lung cancer tends to spread quickly.

Prostate cancer affects men and usually develops slowly, often without noticeable symptoms in the early stages. As the disease progresses, symptoms such as frequent urination, difficulty initiating or stopping urine flow, and blood in the urine may occur. Regular prostate-specific antigen (PSA) screenings are recommended for men over a certain age.

Colorectal cancer can develop in the colon or rectum and often starts as small noncancerous growths called polyps. Symptoms may include changes in bowel habits, blood in the stool, abdominal pain, and unexplained weight loss. Regular screenings, such as colonoscopies, are essential for early detection and removal of polyps before they become cancerous.

Skin cancer, including melanoma, is primarily caused by exposure to ultraviolet (UV) radiation from the sun or tanning beds. It often appears as a new or changing mole, unusual growth, or sore that does not heal. Regular self-examinations and annual dermatological check-ups are vital for detecting skin cancer early.

These are just a few examples of the common types of cancer. It is important to note that early detection and treatment significantly increase the chances of survival and successful outcomes. By being aware of the signs and symptoms associated with different types of cancer, individuals can take a proactive approach to their health and seek medical attention promptly. Regular check-ups, screenings, and self-examinations should be a part of everyone's healthcare routine to ensure timely detection and intervention, potentially saving lives and improving quality of life for those affected by cancer.

Statistics and Prevalence

Cancer is a global health issue that affects millions of individuals every year. In this subchapter, we will delve into the statistics and prevalence of cancer to provide a comprehensive understanding of its impact on society. By shedding light on these facts, we hope to empower individuals to take proactive steps in recognizing signs and symptoms sooner, ultimately leading to earlier detection and improved outcomes.

To truly grasp the magnitude of cancer's prevalence, we must first examine the statistics. According to the World Health Organization (WHO), cancer is the second leading cause of death worldwide, accounting for an estimated 9.6 million deaths in 2018 alone. These numbers are alarming, highlighting the urgent need for increased awareness and early detection efforts.

Furthermore, the American Cancer Society (ACS) reports that approximately 1 in 3 individuals will be diagnosed with cancer at some point in their lives. This means that cancer is an issue that affects all of us, directly or indirectly. It is crucial for everybody to be well-informed about the signs and symptoms, as early detection greatly increases the chances of successful treatment and survival.

When it comes to specific types of cancer, breast cancer is the most prevalent among women, while lung cancer is the leading cause of cancer-related deaths in both men and women. However, it is important to note that cancer can affect anyone, regardless of age, gender, or background. Therefore, a proactive approach to recognizing the signs and symptoms is vital for everyone.

Understanding the prevalence of cancer is just the first step. Armed with this knowledge, individuals can take control of their health and actively seek out information on detecting signs and symptoms sooner. By familiarizing themselves with the warning signs and being proactive in seeking medical advice, individuals can potentially catch cancer at an early stage when treatment options are most effective.

In the next chapters, we will explore specific types of cancer, their unique signs and symptoms, as well as the various screening methods available. By providing comprehensive information and empowering individuals to take action, we aim to equip everyone with the tools they need to detect cancer earlier and increase their chances of successful treatment and survival.

Remember, cancer awareness is not limited to a specific niche but is a crucial subject for everybody. By working together to raise awareness and increase knowledge about cancer, we can make a significant impact in the fight against this devastating disease.

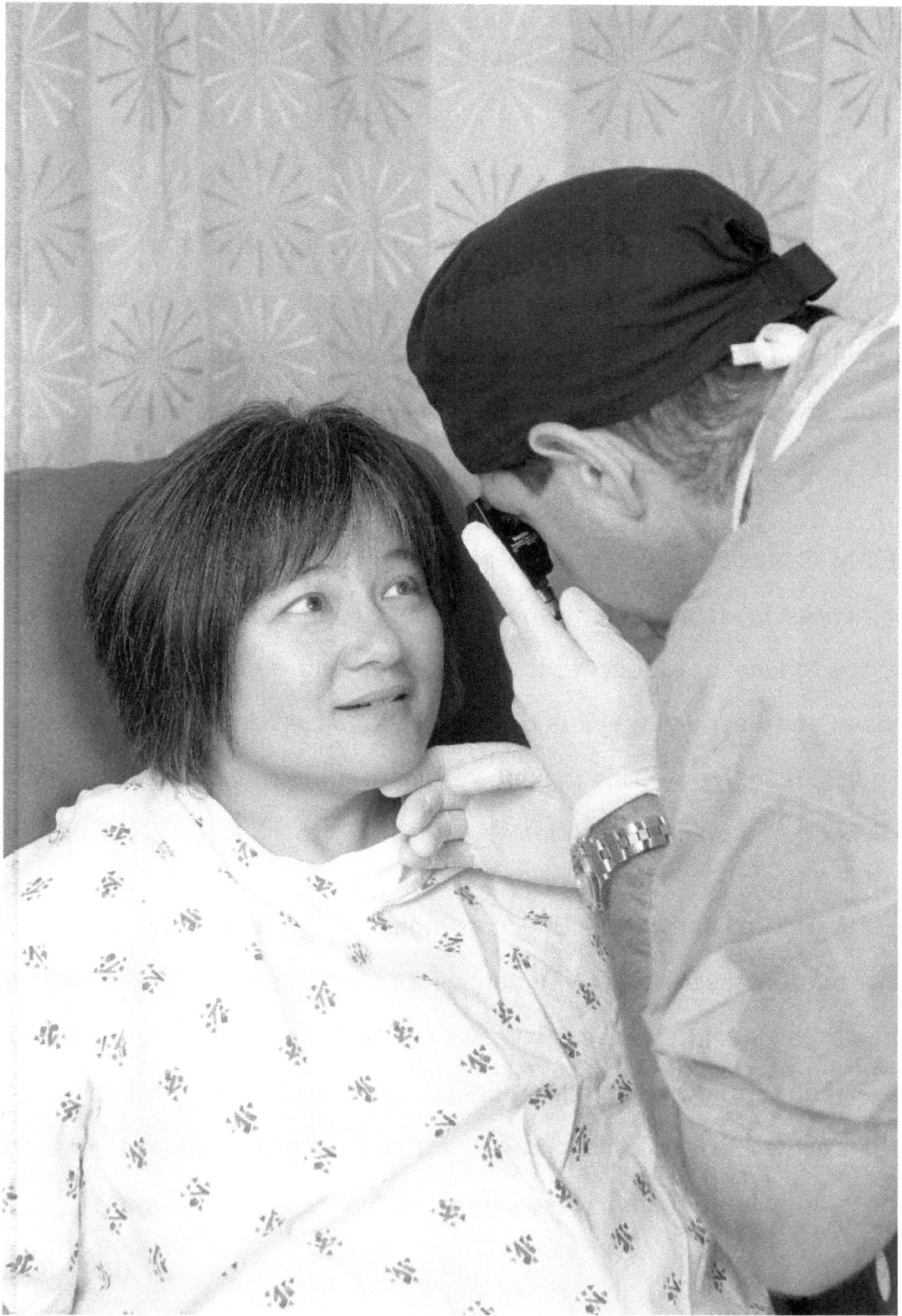

Chapter 2

The Importance of Early Detection

Why Early Detection Matters

In this subchapter, we delve into the critical importance of early detection when it comes to cancer. Cancer is a disease that affects millions of people worldwide, and its impact is far-reaching. However, by understanding why early detection matters, we can empower ourselves to take proactive steps in recognizing the signs and symptoms of cancer sooner.

Early detection plays a pivotal role in improving cancer outcomes. The earlier cancer is detected, the more treatment options are available and the higher the chances of successful treatment and recovery. When cancer is diagnosed at an early stage, it is often more localized and has not yet spread to other parts of the body. This makes treatment more manageable and increases the likelihood of a positive prognosis.

Furthermore, early detection can significantly reduce the emotional and financial burdens associated with cancer. By catching cancer in its early stages, individuals can avoid more invasive and aggressive treatments, resulting in a shorter treatment duration and reduced healthcare costs. Additionally, early detection allows individuals to make informed decisions about their treatment options, empowering them to take charge of their healthcare journey.

For individuals, being aware of the signs and symptoms of cancer is essential. By knowing what to look for, we can detect potential warning signs sooner and seek medical advice promptly. Regular self-examinations, screenings, and understanding our family medical history are all vital components of early detection. Education and awareness are key to ensuring that we can recognize the signs of cancer when they first manifest.

Early detection also benefits society as a whole. By detecting cancer earlier, we can reduce the burden on healthcare systems, allowing for more efficient allocation of medical resources. Additionally, identifying cancer at an early stage can lead to the development of new and improved screening methods, diagnostic tools, and treatment options. The more we understand the importance of early detection, the more we can advocate for research, funding, and policies that support advancements in cancer detection and treatment.

In conclusion, early detection matters. It can save lives, improve treatment outcomes, and alleviate the physical, emotional, and financial burdens associated with cancer. By empowering ourselves with knowledge and being proactive, we can contribute to a society that is better equipped to detect cancer earlier and provide effective treatment options for all.

Benefits of Detecting Cancer Sooner

Early detection of cancer plays a vital role in improving the chances of successful treatment and survival rates. In this subchapter, we will explore the numerous benefits that come with detecting cancer sooner. Understanding these benefits will empower individuals from all walks of life to actively seek out and recognize the signs and symptoms of cancer at an earlier stage.

One of the key advantages of detecting cancer sooner is the increased likelihood of successful treatment. When cancer is detected early, it is often at a localized stage, meaning it has not yet spread to other parts of the body. This allows for more effective treatment options, such as surgery or radiation therapy, which can remove or destroy the cancer cells before they have a chance to metastasize. The earlier the cancer is detected, the higher the chances of complete remission and a positive prognosis.

Another significant benefit is the potential to minimize the impact of treatment on an individual's quality of life. Detecting cancer at an early stage often means that less aggressive treatment options can be utilized, reducing the risk of severe side effects. For example, a small tumor may only require a minimally invasive surgical procedure, sparing the patient from more extensive surgeries or aggressive chemotherapy regimens.

Early detection also allows for the implementation of preventive measures to minimize the risk of cancer recurrence or the development of secondary cancers. By identifying cancer sooner, healthcare professionals can provide patients with targeted counseling and guidance on lifestyle changes, such as dietary modifications, exercise, and smoking cessation, which can significantly reduce the risk of cancer recurrence.

Furthermore, detecting cancer earlier can have a positive impact on healthcare costs. Early-stage cancer treatment tends to be less expensive compared to advanced-stage cancers that require more aggressive interventions. By catching cancer in its early stages, individuals can avoid the financial burden of prolonged and costly treatments.

Lastly, detecting cancer sooner allows individuals to take control of their health and well-being. By being proactive and aware of the signs and symptoms, indiviuals can become their own advocates, seeking medical attention promptly and discussing their concerns with healthcare professionals. Early detection empowers individuals to take charge of their treatment decisions, creating a sense of empowerment and control during a challenging time.

In conclusion, the benefits of detecting cancer sooner are numerous and significant. By understanding the advantages of early detection, individuals from all backgrounds can become more proactive in recognizing the signs and symptoms of cancer. Empowering individuals to take control of their health will ultimately lead to higher survival rates, improved quality of life, reduced healthcare costs, and a greater sense of empowerment for everyone.

CHALLENGES IN EARLY DETECTION

Early detection of cancer is crucial in improving treatment outcomes and saving lives. However, there are several challenges that individuals and healthcare systems face when it comes to recognizing the signs and symptoms of cancer at an early stage. Understanding these challenges can help empower individuals to be more proactive in their own healthcare and raise awareness about the importance of early detection.

One of the main challenges in early detection is the lack of awareness and knowledge about the signs and symptoms of cancer. Many individuals may not know what to look for or may dismiss common symptoms as unrelated to cancer. This lack of awareness can delay diagnosis and treatment, potentially reducing the chances of successful outcomes.

Furthermore, some cancer symptoms can be vague and easily attributed to other less severe conditions. For example, persistent fatigue, unexplained weight loss, or chronic pain can be signs of various health issues, making it difficult to recognize them as potential indicators of cancer. This challenge highlights the need for education and increased awareness among individuals to recognize these symptoms and seek medical attention promptly.

Another significant challenge is the fear and stigma associated with cancer. The fear of a cancer diagnosis can prevent individuals from seeking medical help or delay their decision to undergo screening tests. Additionally, the stigma surrounding cancer can lead to hesitancy in discussing symptoms or concerns with healthcare professionals or even family and friends. Overcoming this challenge involves destigmatizing cancer and promoting open conversations about the disease, encouraging individuals to seek help without fear or judgment.

Moreover, disparities in access to healthcare can pose significant challenges in early detection. Limited access to healthcare facilities, lack of health insurance, or financial constraints can prevent individuals from seeking timely medical attention or undergoing recommended screenings. Addressing these disparities requires a multidimensional approach, including improved access to healthcare services, increased availability of affordable screening programs, and targeted outreach to underserved communities.

In conclusion, early detection of cancer is crucial for improving treatment outcomes, but it is not without its challenges. Lack of awareness, vague symptoms, fear and stigma, and disparities in access to healthcare are some of the key obstacles faced in recognizing cancer signs sooner. By addressing these challenges and empowering individuals with knowledge and resources, we can work towards a future where cancer is detected earlier, leading to more successful treatment and improved survival rates.

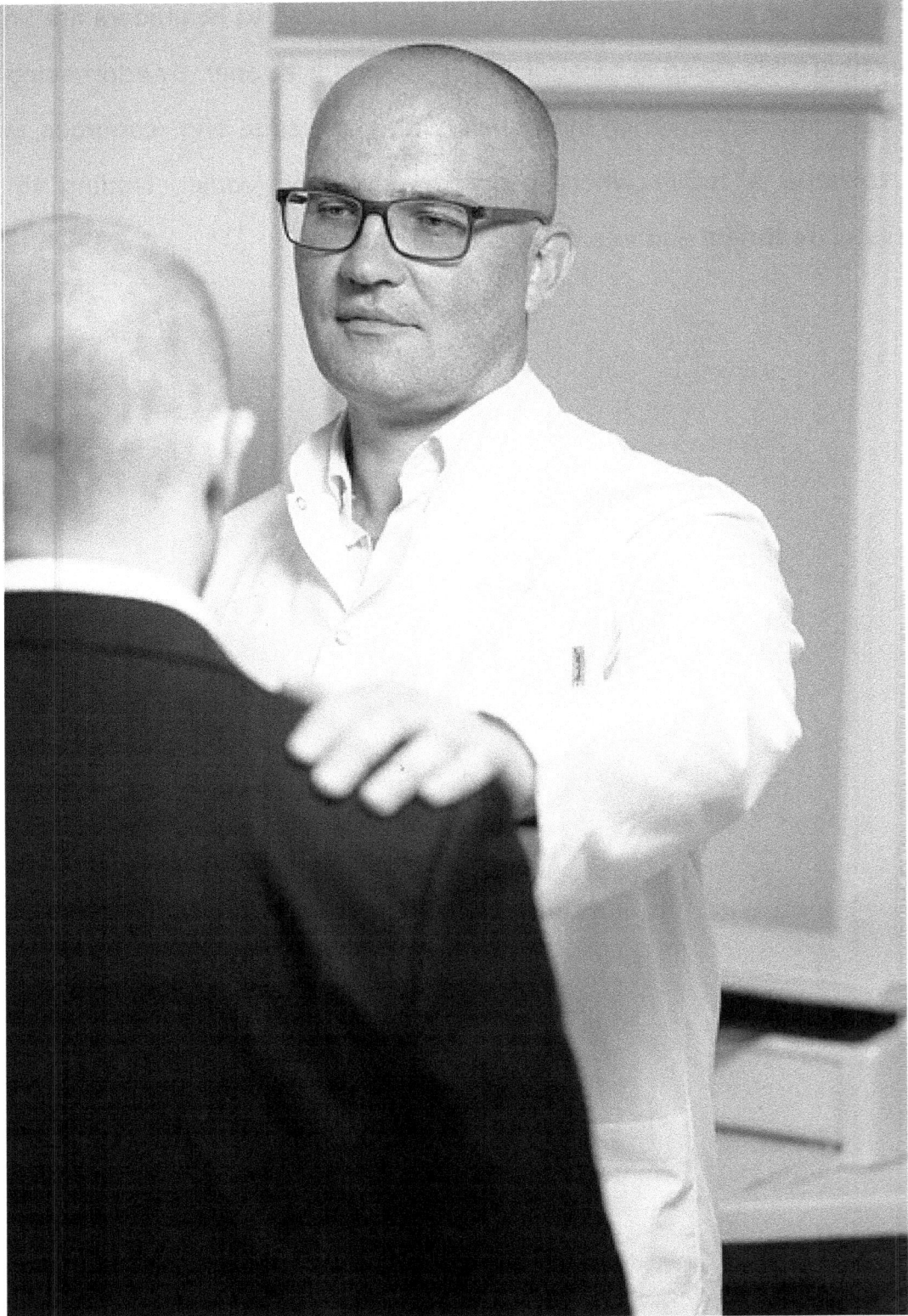

Chapter 3

Common Signs and Symptoms of Cancer

Recognizing General Warning Signs

In our journey towards raising cancer awareness, it is crucial to equip indivicuals from all walks of life with the knowledge and tools to detect cancer signs and symptoms earlier. By recognizing general warning signs, we can empower ourselves and our loved ones to take proactive steps towards early detection and treatment. This subchapter aims to shed light on the general warning signs of cancer that everyone should be aware of.

Cancer can manifest itself in various ways, and while the signs may vary depending on the type and stage of cancer, there are some common warning signs that should not be overlooked. These signs include unexplained weight loss, persistent fatigue, a change in appetite or bowel habits, and unexplained pain or discomfort. It is important to note that these symptoms can be caused by conditions other than cancer, but they should never be ignored.

Furthermore, changes in the skin, such as the appearance of new moles or changes in existing ones, should not be disregarded. Additionally, any unusual bleeding or discharge, whether it is from the rectum, bladder, or any other part of the body, should be promptly addressed. Lastly, the presence of persistent coughing, hoarseness, or difficulty swallowing should not be taken lightly, as they can be indicative of underlying issues, including cancer.

By recognizing these general warning signs, we can become more attuned to our bodies and take appropriate action. It is essential to consult a healthcare professional if any of these symptoms persist for an extended period or if they significantly affect our day-to-day lives. Remember, early detection significantly increases the chances of successful treatment and recovery.

In this subchapter, we will delve deeper into each of these warning signs, exploring their potential causes and when to seek medical attention. We will also provide practical tips on self-examinations and when to schedule regular screenings. Additionally, we will address the importance of maintaining a healthy lifestyle, including exercise, proper nutrition, and stress management, as these factors play a crucial role in cancer prevention.

By empowering ourselves with knowledge and recognizing general warning signs, we can become proactive in our approach to cancer detection. Together, let us spread awareness and equip individuals from all walks of life with the tools to detect cancer signs sooner and ultimately save lives. Remember, early detection is key, and by being vigilant, we can make a difference in the fight against cancer.

Specific Symptoms for Different Types of Cancer

When it comes to cancer, early detection is crucial for successful treatment and improved outcomes. Recognizing the signs and symptoms associated with various types of cancer can empower individuals to take proactive steps towards their health. In this subchapter, we will explore the specific symptoms that may indicate the presence of different types of cancer, providing valuable knowledge to everyone.

Lung cancer, one of the most common types worldwide, often presents symptoms like persistent cough, chest pain, shortness of breath, and coughing up blood. Breast cancer, predominantly affecting women, can manifest as a lump or thickening in the breast or underarm area, changes in breast size or shape, nipple discharge, or redness and dimpling of the skin. Prostate cancer, typically affecting men, may show symptoms such as frequent urination, weak urine flow, blood in urine or semen, or discomfort in the pelvic area.

Colon cancer symptoms may include changes in bowel movements like persistent diarrhea or constipation, rectal bleeding, abdominal pain, and unexplained weight loss. Skin cancer, the most common type of cancer, often exhibits warning signs such as changes in the size, shape, or color of a mole, the appearance of new growths, or a sore that does not heal.

Recognizing symptoms of ovarian cancer is crucial, as it is often diagnosed at an advanced stage. Symptoms may include abdominal bloating, pelvic pain, frequent urination, fatigue, and changes in appetite. Pancreatic cancer symptoms include jaundice, unexplained weight loss, abdominal or back pain, and digestive issues.

Other types of cancer, such as cervical, bladder, kidney, and leukemia, also have unique symptoms that individuals should be aware of. By familiarizing themselves with these specific symptoms, individuals can be proactive in seeking medical attention when necessary, potentially leading to earlier diagnosis and better treatment outcomes.

Remember, these symptoms are not definitive proof of cancer. However, they serve as red flags, indicating the need for further investigation by a healthcare professional. Early detection offers a greater chance of successful treatment and recovery.

In conclusion, being aware of the specific symptoms associated with different types of cancer is essential for everyone. By educating ourselves about the warning signs and taking prompt action, we can empower ourselves and our loved ones to detect cancer earlier. This subchapter serves as a proactive guide, equipping individuals with the knowledge they need to recognize signs and symptoms sooner, thus promoting a proactive approach towards cancer awareness and prevention.

Understanding the Variability in Symptoms

When it comes to cancer, understanding the variability in symptoms is crucial for early detection and timely treatment. Cancer is a complex disease that can affect different parts of the body, and its symptoms can vary widely from person to person. This subchapter aims to shed light on this variability, empowering everybody to recognize the signs sooner.

One of the reasons for the variability in symptoms is the type and stage of cancer. Different types of cancer have different characteristic symptoms. For example, lung cancer often presents with persistent cough, shortness of breath, and chest pain, while breast cancer may manifest as a lump or changes in the breast's shape or texture. Additionally, the stage of cancer, which indicates how far the disease has progressed, plays a role in symptom variation. Early-stage cancer may have mild or no symptoms at all, making it harder to detect.

Another factor contributing to variability is the individual's unique genetic makeup and overall health. Each person's body can react differently to cancer cells, leading to a wide range of symptoms. Additionally, existing medical conditions or lifestyle choices, such as smoking or exposure to certain chemicals, can influence the manifestation of cancer symptoms.

It is important to note that cancer symptoms can also mimic other, less severe conditions. For instance, fatigue and weight loss, common symptoms of various cancers, can also be attributed to stress or other illnesses. This makes it essential for individuals to pay attention to persistent or unusual symptoms that do not resolve with time or conventional treatment.

To better understand the variability in symptoms, it is crucial to be aware of the "red flags" that may indicate cancer. These include unexplained weight loss, persistent pain, changes in the skin, unusual bleeding or discharge, and persistent fatigue. By being vigilant and recognizing these warning signs, individuals can take a proactive approach towards their health and seek medical attention when necessary.

In conclusion, understanding the variability in symptoms is key to detecting cancer earlier. By familiarizing ourselves with the different types of cancer and their symptoms, paying attention to our bodies, and recognizing the "red flags," we can empower ourselves to take control of our health. This subchapter aims to provide the necessary knowledge to help everybody become more aware and proactive in recognizing the signs and symptoms of cancer sooner.

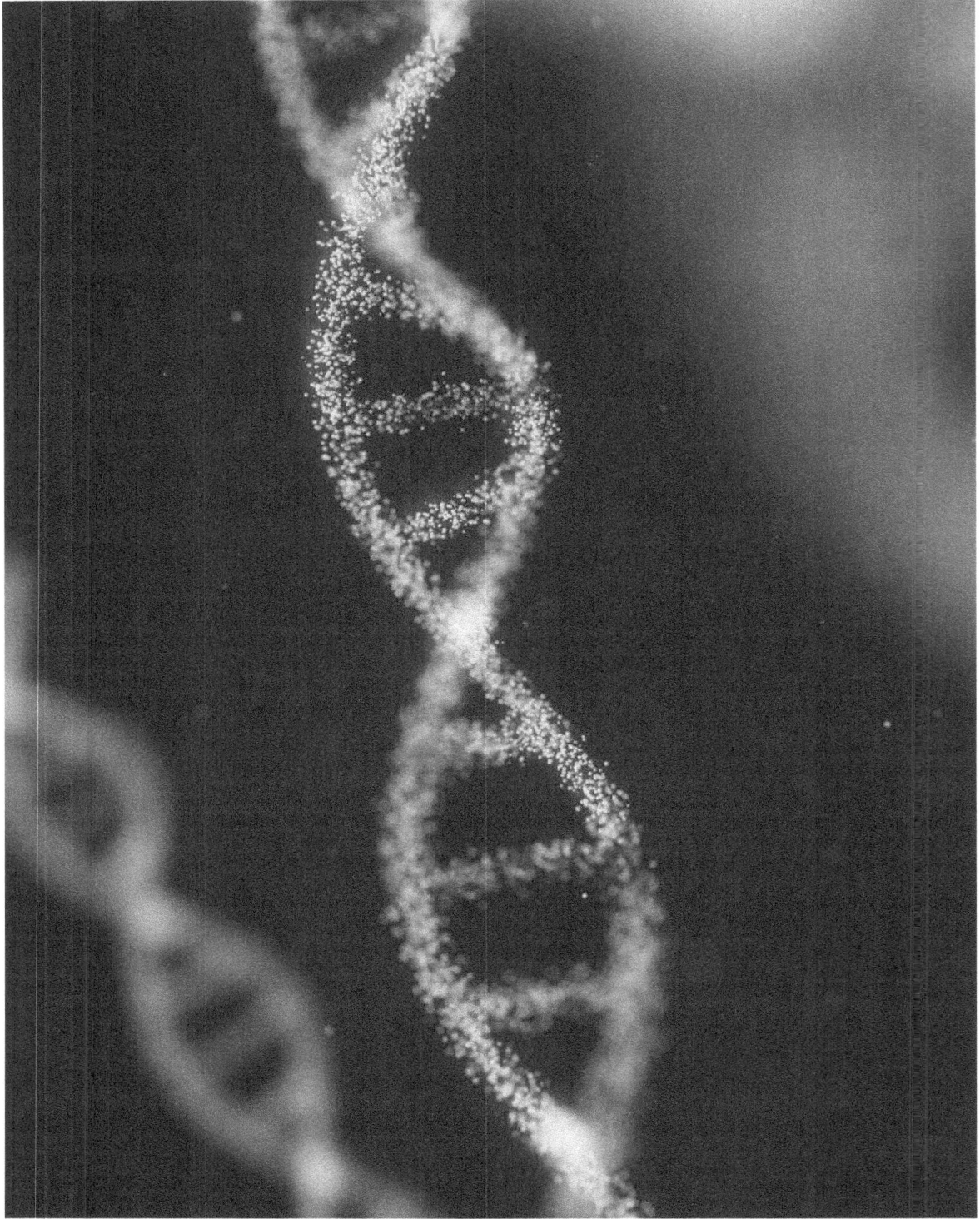

Chapter 4

Risk Factors and Prevention Strategies

Genetic and Hereditary Factors

Understanding the role of genetic and hereditary factors in cancer development is crucial in our journey towards early detection and prevention. While cancer can affect anyone, regardless of their genetic background, it is essential to acknowledge that certain individuals may have a higher risk due to inherited gene mutations. In this subchapter, we will explore the significance of genetic and hereditary factors in cancer and how they can influence our proactive approach to recognizing signs and symptoms sooner.

Genetic factors refer to the genes we inherit from our parents. These genes carry instructions for our cells' growth, division, and repair. Sometimes, mutations or changes occur in these genes, which can increase the likelihood of developing cancer. Hereditary factors, on the other hand, involve the passing down of these mutated genes from one generation to another. This hereditary transmission can significantly impact an individual's predisposition to certain types of cancer.

One of the most well-known examples of hereditary cancer is breast and ovarian cancer caused by mutations in the BRCA1 and BRCA2 genes. Individuals carrying these gene mutations have a higher risk of developing these types of cancer compared to the general population. Genetic testing can help identify these mutations and enable individuals to take proactive measures, such as increased surveillance or preventive surgeries, to reduce their risk.

It is important to note that not all gene mutations directly result in cancer. Some mutations may increase the risk but do not guarantee the development of the disease. Other factors, such as lifestyle choices and environmental exposures, play a significant role in determining whether or not cancer will manifest.

Understanding our genetic and hereditary factors can empower us to make informed decisions about our health. Genetic counseling and testing can provide valuable insights into our individual risk profiles, guiding us towards appropriate actions for early detection and prevention. By identifying high-risk individuals, healthcare providers can offer personalized screening plans, allowing for the detection of cancer at its earliest and most treatable stages.

In conclusion, genetic and hereditary factors contribute to the development and risk of cancer. Acknowledging and understanding these factors can help us take a proactive approach to recognize signs and symptoms sooner. By combining genetic testing, counseling, and lifestyle modifications, we can empower ourselves to detect cancer earlier, leading to improved outcomes and a higher chance of survival. Remember, knowledge is power, and by arming ourselves with information about our genetic and hereditary factors, we can take control of our health and well-being.

Lifestyle and Environmental Risk Factors

In our quest to understand cancer and empower individuals to detect signs sooner, it is essential to explore the role of lifestyle and environmental risk factors. While genetics certainly play a significant part in cancer development, it is crucial to acknowledge that many cases of cancer are preventable through lifestyle modifications and environmental awareness. By recognizing these risk factors, we can take proactive steps towards minimizing our chances of developing cancer.

One of the most prominent lifestyle risk factors associated with cancer is tobacco use. Smoking cigarettes, cigars, or pipes is directly linked to several types of cancer, including lung, throat, and mouth cancers. Additionally, exposure to secondhand smoke can also increase the risk. By quitting smoking or avoiding exposure to secondhand smoke, we can significantly reduce our chances of developing these types of cancer.

Another lifestyle factor that has gained attention in recent years is the role of diet and physical activity. A diet rich in fruits, vegetables, whole grains, and lean proteins has been associated with a decreased risk of several types of cancer. On the other hand, a diet high in processed foods, red meats, and unhealthy fats may increase the risk. Regular physical activity is also crucial, as it helps maintain a healthy weight and reduces the risk of certain cancers, such as breast and colon cancer.

Environmental risk factors are equally important to consider. Exposure to certain chemicals and pollutants in our surroundings can significantly increase the risk of cancer. For instance, prolonged exposure to asbestos, radon, and certain industrial chemicals has been linked to lung cancer. Similarly, exposure to UV radiation from the sun or tanning beds increases the risk of skin cancer. By being aware of these environmental risk factors and taking necessary precautions, such as wearing protective clothing and using sunscreen, we can minimize our exposure and reduce the risk of cancer.

In conclusion, lifestyle and environmental risk factors play a critical role in cancer development. By being proactive and making conscious choices, we can significantly reduce our chances of developing cancer. Quitting smoking, adopting a healthy diet and regular exercise routine, and staying aware of environmental risks are all steps towards a healthier and cancer-free future. Let us empower ourselves with knowledge and take charge of our lifestyles to detect cancer signs sooner and live a life free from this devastating disease.

Preventive Measures and Healthy Habits

In this subchapter, we will explore the importance of preventive measures and healthy habits in the context of cancer awareness. By adopting these practices, individuals can empower themselves to detect signs of cancer earlier, leading to better chances of successful treatment and improved outcomes. Whether you have a family history of cancer or not, everyone can benefit from these proactive strategies.

One of the most crucial preventive measures is to undergo regular screenings. These screenings can vary depending on the type of cancer and your age group, but they play a vital role in early detection. Regular mammograms for breast cancer, pap smears for cervical cancer, and colonoscopies for colorectal cancer are just a few examples of screenings that can help identify potential issues before symptoms develop. By prioritizing these screenings and following the recommended schedules, individuals can catch cancer in its early stages when it is most treatable.

Another important aspect of preventive measures is understanding and managing risk factors. By identifying personal risk factors such as smoking, excessive alcohol consumption, poor diet, lack of physical activity, and exposure to carcinogens, individuals can take proactive steps to mitigate these risks. For example, quitting smoking, reducing alcohol intake, adopting a healthy diet rich in fruits and vegetables, and engaging in regular exercise can significantly lower the chances of developing cancer.

Beyond preventive measures, cultivating healthy habits can also contribute to cancer awareness. Being aware of your body and paying attention to any changes or unusual symptoms is critical. Regular self-examinations, such as breast self-exams or skin checks, can help individuals detect any abnormalities early on. Additionally, staying informed about the signs and symptoms of different types of cancer can empower individuals to seek medical attention promptly if they notice anything concerning.

Incorporating healthy habits into your lifestyle is not only beneficial for cancer prevention but also for overall well-being. A balanced diet, regular exercise, stress management, and adequate sleep are all essential for maintaining a healthy immune system and reducing the risk of cancer. By making these habits a priority, individuals can enhance their body's natural defenses against cancer and other diseases.

Preventive measures and healthy habits are crucial for cancer awareness and early detection. By adopting these practices, individuals can take charge of their health and significantly improve their chances of catching cancer in its early stages. Remember, it is never too early to start implementing these habits, and it is never too late to make positive changes for a healthier future.

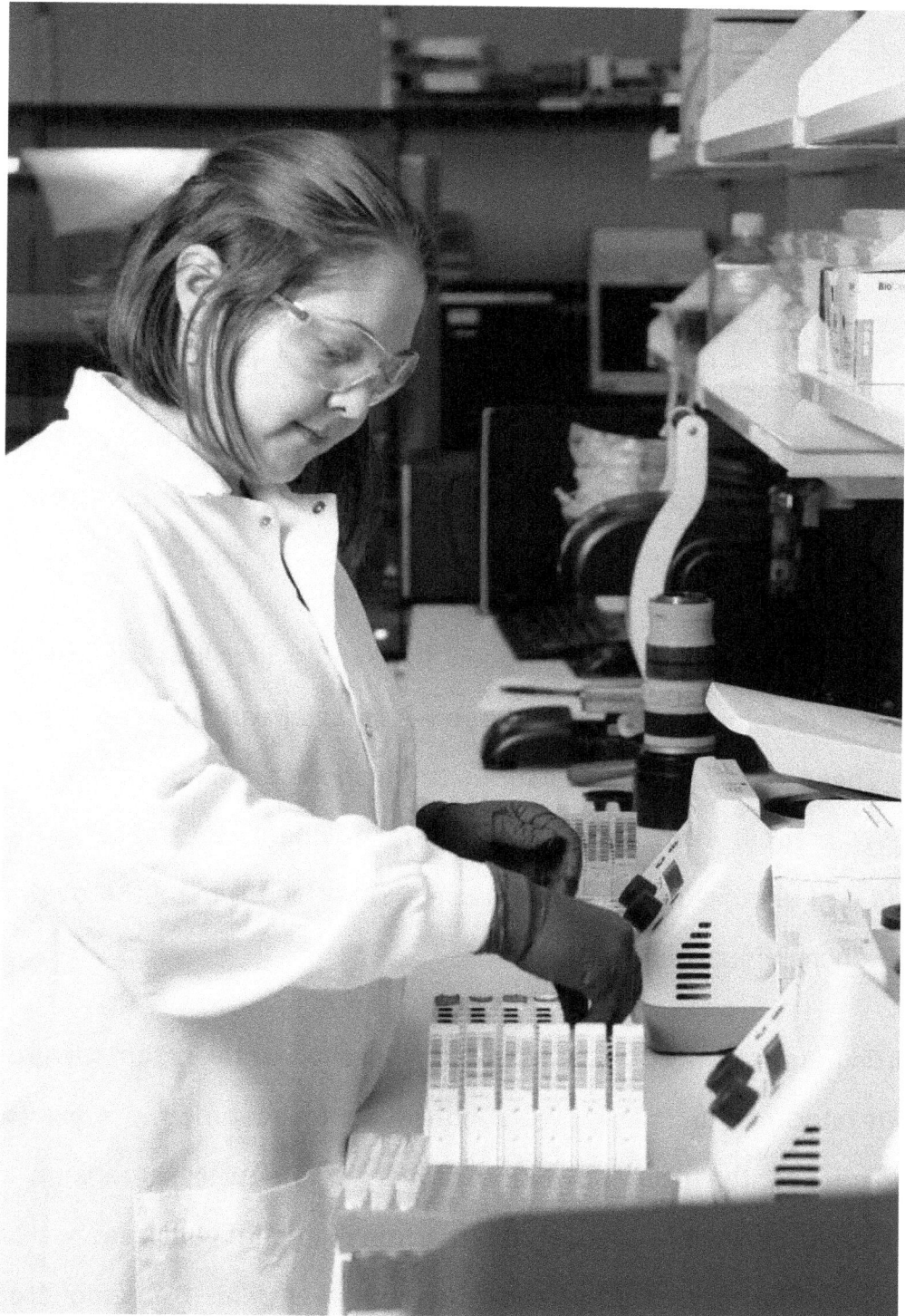

Chapter 5

Screening and Diagnostic Tests

Understanding Screening Programs

Screening programs play a crucial role in the early detection and prevention of cancer. By participating in these programs, individuals can increase their chances of detecting the signs and symptoms of cancer at an early stage when treatment options are more effective. This subchapter aims to provide a comprehensive understanding of screening programs, their importance, and how they can empower individuals to detect signs of cancer sooner.

Screening programs are designed to identify individuals who may be at higher risk of developing cancer or those who may already have early signs of the disease. These programs utilize various tests and examinations to detect cancer in its early stages, even before symptoms manifest. By doing so, screening programs can significantly improve survival rates and reduce the overall impact of cancer on individuals and society.

Participating in a screening program is a proactive step towards taking control of one's health. It empowers individuals to become more aware of their own bodies and the potential signs of cancer. Regular screenings can help identify any abnormalities or changes that may indicate the presence of cancer, prompting further investigation and potential treatment. By being proactive in their approach, individuals can increase their chances of detecting cancer earlier, when it is more treatable.

It is important to note that different types of cancer have different screening recommendations. For instance, breast cancer screenings often involve mammograms, while colorectal cancer screenings may include colonoscopies or stool tests. Understanding the specific screening recommendations for different types of cancer is essential for individuals to make informed decisions about their health.

Screening programs also benefit society as a whole. By detecting cancer at an early stage, healthcare providers can intervene promptly, potentially preventing the disease from progressing or spreading. This, in turn, reduces the burden on healthcare systems and improves overall public health.

In conclusion, understanding screening programs is vital for everybody. By participating in these programs, individuals can empower themselves to detect signs of cancer sooner, leading to earlier intervention, improved treatment outcomes, and increased survival rates. Regular screenings, tailored to specific cancer types, enable individuals to take control of their health and become proactive in the fight against cancer. Ultimately, screening programs not only benefit individuals but also contribute to a healthier society as a whole.

Common Diagnostic Tests

In the battle against cancer, early detection is crucial. The sooner cancer is detected, the more effective the treatment options become, and the better the chances of survival. This subchapter aims to educate everybody on the common diagnostic tests used to detect cancer, empowering individuals to recognize signs and symptoms sooner.

One of the most frequently used diagnostic tests is a biopsy. This involves the removal of a small sample of tissue from the suspected area. The sample is then examined under a microscope to determine if cancerous cells are present. Biopsies can be performed through various methods, including needle biopsies, surgical biopsies, or even liquid biopsies, which detect cancer cells or DNA fragments circulating in the blood.

Another common diagnostic test is imaging techniques, such as X-rays, CT scans, MRIs, and ultrasounds. These non-invasive tests allow medical professionals to visualize the internal structures of the body, identifying any abnormal growths, tumors, or masses. These imaging tests are particularly useful in identifying the location and size of tumors, aiding in the diagnosis and staging of cancer.

Blood tests are also widely utilized in cancer detection. These tests measure various substances in the blood that may indicate the presence of cancer, such as tumor markers or specific proteins produced by cancer cells. Although blood tests alone cannot diagnose cancer, they provide valuable information that prompts further investigation.

For certain types of cancer, screening tests are recommended for early detection in individuals without symptoms. Mammograms, for example, are used to screen for breast cancer in women, while Pap tests are used to screen for cervical cancer in women. Other screening tests include colonoscopies for colorectal cancer and PSA tests for prostate cancer in men.

Furthermore, genetic testing plays an essential role in identifying individuals who may have an inherited predisposition to certain types of cancer. These tests analyze DNA to identify specific gene mutations associated with an increased risk of developing cancer. Early knowledge of genetic predispositions can allow for proactive measures and more frequent screening to catch cancer at its earliest stages.

By familiarizing ourselves with these common diagnostic tests, we can take a proactive approach to our health and be better equipped to recognize the signs and symptoms of cancer sooner. Remember, early detection saves lives, and everyone can play a vital role in the fight against cancer by staying informed and taking action.

WHEN AND HOW OFTEN SHOULD YOU GET SCREENED?

Regular cancer screenings are crucial for early detection and treatment. The timing and frequency of these screenings can vary depending on various factors. In this subchapter, we will explore the recommended guidelines for cancer screenings to empower individuals in detecting signs sooner.

The timing of cancer screenings can be influenced by age, gender, family history, and lifestyle choices. For instance, women should start getting regular mammograms around the age of 40 or earlier if they have a family history of breast cancer. Similarly, men and women should undergo regular colonoscopies starting at the age of 50, or earlier if they have a family history of colorectal cancer. It is essential to consult with your healthcare provider to determine the appropriate age to begin screenings for specific cancers.

The frequency of screenings also depends on various factors. Some screenings are recommended annually, while others may be done every few years. For example, Pap smears, which detect cervical cancer, are typically conducted every three years for women aged 21 to 65. Prostate-specific antigen (PSA) tests for prostate cancer may be done annually for men over the age of 50. However, these guidelines are not set in stone, and individual circumstances may require more frequent or earlier screenings.

Furthermore, it is crucial for individuals to be aware of their own bodies and be proactive. If you notice any unusual changes or symptoms that persist, regardless of your age or gender, it is essential to consult with your healthcare provider. Early detection can significantly increase the chances of successful treatment.

It is important to note that these guidelines are general recommendations, and your healthcare provider may suggest different screening schedules based on your individual risk factors and medical history. Additionally, advancements in medical research and technology may lead to updates in screening guidelines. Staying informed about the latest recommendations is vital to ensure you are receiving the most effective screenings for early cancer detection.

In conclusion, regular cancer screenings are crucial for everyone, regardless of age or gender. Following the recommended guidelines and being proactive about your health can help detect cancer signs sooner, increasing the likelihood of successful treatment. Consult with your healthcare provider to determine the appropriate timing and frequency of screenings based on your individual risk factors and medical history. Remember, early detection saves lives.

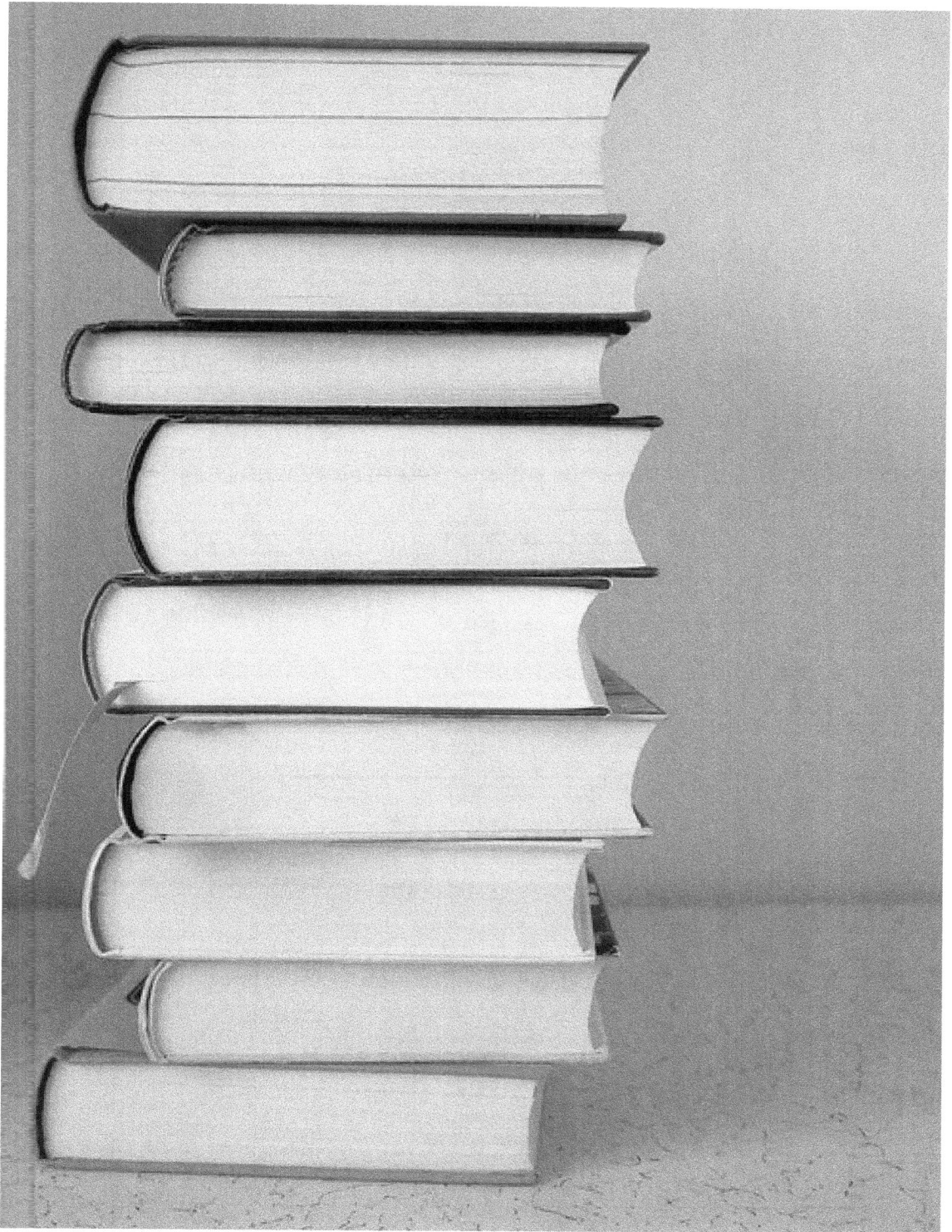

CHAPTER 6

EMPOWERING INDIVIDUALS FOR EARLY DETECTION

CREATING AWARENESS AND EDUCATION

In the fight against cancer, knowledge is power. It is essential to empower individuals with the tools they need to detect signs and symptoms sooner, as early detection is often the key to successful treatment and improved outcomes. This subchapter, titled "Creating Awareness and Education," aims to provide a comprehensive guide for everybody interested in learning how to discover cancer earlier.

The first step towards creating awareness is understanding the importance of regular screenings and self-examinations. By educating individuals about the various types of cancer and their warning signs, we can encourage a proactive approach to healthcare. This section will delve into the specific signs and symptoms associated with different types of cancer, equipping readers with the knowledge needed to identify potential red flags.

Additionally, this subchapter will explore the significance of lifestyle choices in cancer prevention. By adopting a healthy lifestyle, individuals can significantly reduce their risk of developing certain types of cancer. Topics such as maintaining a balanced diet, engaging in regular physical activity, managing stress, and avoiding tobacco and excessive alcohol consumption will be discussed in detail.

Furthermore, creating awareness and education requires addressing the myths, misconceptions, and stigmas surrounding cancer. By debunking common misconceptions and providing accurate information, we can foster a more supportive and understanding environment for cancer patients and survivors. This subchapter will explore the importance of empathy, compassion, and open dialogue when discussing cancer-related topics.

To effectively spread awareness, this section will also address the role of media, community organizations, and healthcare professionals in disseminating information. It will highlight the significance of educational campaigns, social media platforms, and support groups in reaching a wider audience and providing resources for individuals seeking information or support.

Ultimately, the goal of this subchapter is to empower individuals to take control of their health by recognizing the signs and symptoms of cancer earlier. By promoting education and awareness, we can contribute to a society that is better equipped to detect and combat this devastating disease. Whether you are a healthcare professional, a concerned family member, or an individual interested in safeguarding your own well-being, the information presented in this subchapter will prove invaluable in your journey towards cancer awareness and prevention.

Self-Examination Techniques

In the battle against cancer, early detection plays a vital role in increasing the chances of successful treatment and recovery. This subchapter aims to empower everybody with self-examination techniques that can help detect signs of cancer sooner. By familiarizing yourself with these techniques, you become an active participant in your own health, enabling you to recognize potential symptoms at an early stage.

Breast self-examination is a crucial technique for early detection of breast cancer. By conducting regular self-exams, both men and women can identify any changes in their breast tissue. This simple procedure involves carefully examining the breasts for lumps, changes in size or shape, and any unusual discharge. It is recommended to perform breast self-exams once a month, ideally a few days after the menstrual cycle ends.

Another important self-examination technique is the skin check. Skin cancer is one of the most common forms of cancer, and early detection significantly improves the chances of successful treatment. Regularly inspecting your skin for any changes in moles, freckles, or new growths is crucial. Use a mirror to examine hard-to-see areas and pay close attention to any changes in color, shape, or size. If you notice any suspicious changes, consult a healthcare professional immediately.

Oral cancer is another condition that can be detected through self-examination. By regularly inspecting your mouth, gums, tongue, and throat for any unusual sores, lumps, or discoloration, you can catch potential signs of oral cancer earlier. If you spot anything out of the ordinary, schedule an appointment with your dentist or doctor promptly.

Beyond these specific techniques, it is important to cultivate a general awareness of your body and its functioning. Pay attention to any persistent changes, such as unexplained weight loss, chronic fatigue, or prolonged pain. These symptoms may indicate an underlying health issue, including various types of cancer. By being attuned to your body, you can recognize potential warning signs and seek medical attention promptly.

Remember, early detection is key in the fight against cancer. By practicing self-examination techniques and maintaining a vigilant attitude towards your health, you can increase the likelihood of catching cancer at its early stages, greatly improving the chances of successful treatment and recovery. Empower yourself with knowledge and take control of your health today.

Encouraging Regular Check-ups and Doctor Visits

Regular check-ups and doctor visits are essential for maintaining good health and detecting any signs of cancer early on. In this subchapter, we will explore the importance of these routine visits and how they can empower individuals to detect signs of cancer sooner.

Visiting your doctor on a regular basis is crucial for several reasons. Firstly, it allows you to establish a strong relationship with your healthcare provider, who can become familiar with your medical history, lifestyle, and any potential risk factors for cancer. This relationship enables your doctor to better identify any changes or symptoms that may be indicative of cancer.

Another key benefit of regular check-ups is the opportunity for preventive screenings. These screenings can detect cancer in its earliest stages, when treatment is often more effective. Depending on your age, gender, and family history, your doctor may recommend screenings such as mammograms, pap smears, colonoscopies, and prostate exams. By undergoing these screenings at the recommended intervals, you increase your chances of detecting cancer at an early and treatable stage.

Furthermore, regular check-ups provide an opportunity for health education and awareness. Your doctor can provide you with valuable information about cancer prevention, lifestyle modifications, and self-examination techniques. They can also address any concerns or questions you may have, ultimately empowering you to take a proactive approach to your health.

It is important to remember that regular check-ups are not limited to physical examinations. Mental health plays a crucial role in overall well-being, and discussing any emotional or psychological concerns with your doctor is equally important. Cancer can have a significant impact on mental health, and early detection and intervention can make a world of difference.

In conclusion, encouraging regular check-ups and doctor visits is imperative for everyone. By establishing a strong relationship with your healthcare provider, undergoing preventive screenings, and staying informed about cancer prevention, you are taking proactive steps towards detecting signs of cancer sooner. Remember, early detection is key to increasing treatment success rates and ultimately saving lives.

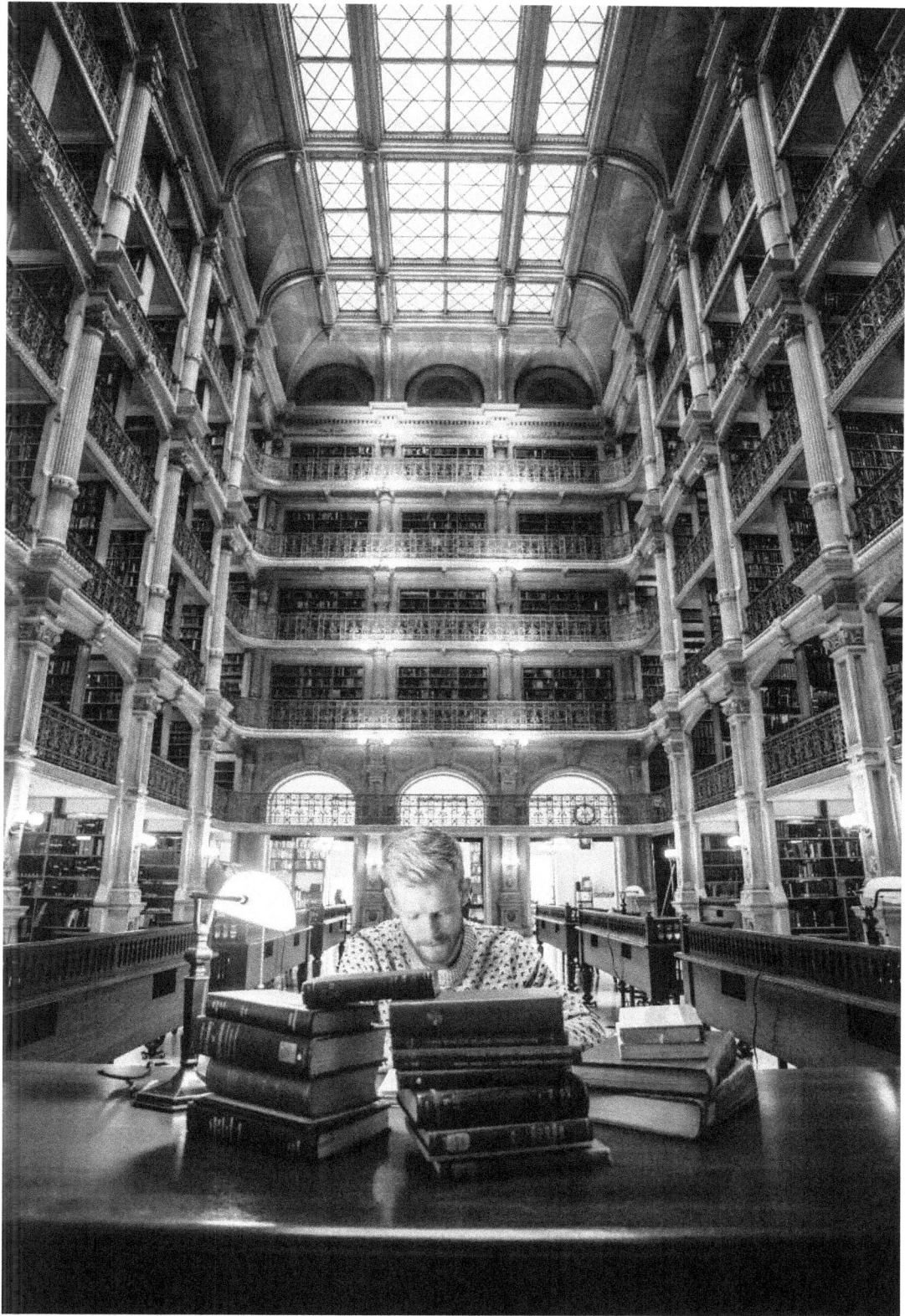

Chapter 7

Support and Resources for Cancer Detection

Accessing Support Networks

When faced with a cancer diagnosis, it is crucial for individuals to have a strong support system in place. This subchapter explores the importance of accessing support networks and the various resources available to individuals and their loved ones during their cancer journey.

Cancer can be a daunting and overwhelming experience, both physically and emotionally. However, nobody has to face it alone. Support networks play a vital role in providing comfort, guidance, and encouragement to those affected by cancer. By reaching out to others, individuals can find solace in shared experiences, gain valuable advice, and access a wealth of resources tailored to their specific needs.

There are numerous avenues to access support networks when dealing with cancer. One of the first steps is to inform family and friends about the diagnosis. Loved ones can provide emotional support, accompany individuals to medical appointments, and lend a helping hand during treatment. Additionally, joining cancer support groups can connect individuals with others who are going through similar experiences. These groups offer a safe space to share feelings, exchange information, and learn coping strategies.

Healthcare professionals are also an essential part of the support network. Oncologists, nurses, and social workers are trained to provide guidance and support throughout the cancer journey. They can offer information on treatment options, help manage side effects, and connect individuals with relevant support services such as counseling or financial assistance.

In addition to personal networks and healthcare professionals, there are numerous organizations and online platforms dedicated to supporting individuals affected by cancer. These resources provide information on various types of cancer, treatment options, and survivorship. They may also offer helplines, online forums, and educational materials to address specific concerns. Some organizations even provide financial aid or help individuals navigate insurance and healthcare systems.

Remember, accessing support networks is not a sign of weakness but a sign of strength. By reaching out to others, individuals can find the support they need to navigate the challenges of cancer and improve their overall well-being. Empowering oneself with knowledge, connecting with others, and seeking support are essential steps towards detecting signs and symptoms of cancer sooner, improving treatment outcomes, and enhancing the quality of life for everyone impacted by this disease.

Utilizing Online Resources and Tools

In today's digital age, the internet has become an invaluable resource for accessing information and connecting with others. When it comes to cancer awareness and early detection, online resources and tools can play a crucial role in empowering individuals to recognize signs and symptoms sooner. This subchapter explores the various ways in which everyone can utilize online platforms to enhance their understanding of cancer and take proactive steps towards detection.

One of the key benefits of online resources is the wealth of information available at our fingertips. Websites, blogs, and online forums dedicated to cancer awareness provide a comprehensive range of knowledge, from understanding different types of cancer to learning about the latest advancements in treatment. By exploring these resources, individuals can educate themselves about the warning signs, risk factors, and preventive measures associated with various types of cancer.

Moreover, online tools can assist individuals in assessing their own risk factors and monitoring their health. Many websites offer interactive quizzes and questionnaires that help determine an individual's susceptibility to certain types of cancer. Additionally, online platforms enable users to track their symptoms, schedule regular check-ups, and set reminders for routine screenings. These tools not only facilitate early detection but also encourage individuals to take an active role in their healthcare.

Online communities and support networks also play a vital role in cancer awareness. Social media platforms and online forums provide spaces where individuals can connect with others who have experienced similar situations. These communities offer a safe environment for sharing personal stories, seeking advice, and finding emotional support. By joining these networks, individuals can gain insights, learn about coping strategies, and find solace in knowing they are not alone in their journey.

Furthermore, online platforms have revolutionized the way individuals can access professional medical advice. Telemedicine services allow people to consult with healthcare professionals remotely, reducing the need for physical appointments. This accessibility is particularly beneficial for individuals in remote areas or those with mobility limitations. By leveraging these resources, individuals can seek expert guidance, clarify doubts, and receive timely advice without leaving their homes.

In conclusion, the internet and online resources have transformed the way we approach cancer awareness and early detection. By utilizing these tools, individuals can educate themselves, assess their risk factors, monitor their health, connect with others, and seek professional advice. Empowering everyone with knowledge and support, online resources play a pivotal role in detecting signs and symptoms sooner, ultimately leading to better outcomes in the fight against cancer.

Engaging with Healthcare Professionals

When it comes to detecting and managing cancer, engaging with healthcare professionals is crucial. These dedicated individuals possess the knowledge, skills, and resources to guide you through the complex journey of cancer awareness, diagnosis, and treatment. In this subchapter, we will explore the various ways you can effectively engage with healthcare professionals to empower yourself and detect cancer signs sooner.

First and foremost, it is essential to establish a strong partnership with your primary care physician. Regular check-ups and open communication are key to maintaining your overall health. During these visits, share any concerns or symptoms you may have, even if they seem minor. Your physician can conduct the necessary screenings and tests to detect any signs of cancer at an early stage.

Additionally, it is vital to be an active participant in your healthcare journey. Educate yourself about the common signs and symptoms of different types of cancer, as outlined in our book, "How to Discover Cancer Earlier: A Proactive Guide to Recognizing Signs and Symptoms Sooner." By familiarizing yourself with these signs, you can better communicate with your healthcare professionals and provide them with valuable information that may lead to an early diagnosis.

Another valuable resource for engaging with healthcare professionals is support groups and patient advocacy organizations. These groups offer a platform for individuals affected by cancer to share experiences, gain knowledge, and access support networks. By joining such groups, you can connect with people who have gone through similar experiences and learn from their journeys. These interactions can also provide insights into the medical professionals and facilities that have made a positive impact on others' cancer detection and treatment.

When engaging with healthcare professionals, be sure to ask questions and seek clarification whenever necessary. It is your right to fully understand your diagnosis, treatment options, and potential side effects. By actively participating in the decision-making process, you can make informed choices that align with your personal values and preferences.

Lastly, remember that engaging with healthcare professionals is not limited to the duration of your treatment. It is essential to maintain regular follow-up appointments, even after successful treatment or remission. These visits will help monitor your progress, detect any potential recurrence, and ensure your long-term well-being.

n conclusion, engaging with healthcare professionals is a crucial aspect of cancer awareness and detection. By establishing strong relationships with your primary care physician, educating yourself, joining support groups, and actively participating in your healthcare journey, you can empower yourself to detect cancer signs sooner. Remember, early detection can save lives, and together, we can make a difference in the fight against cancer.

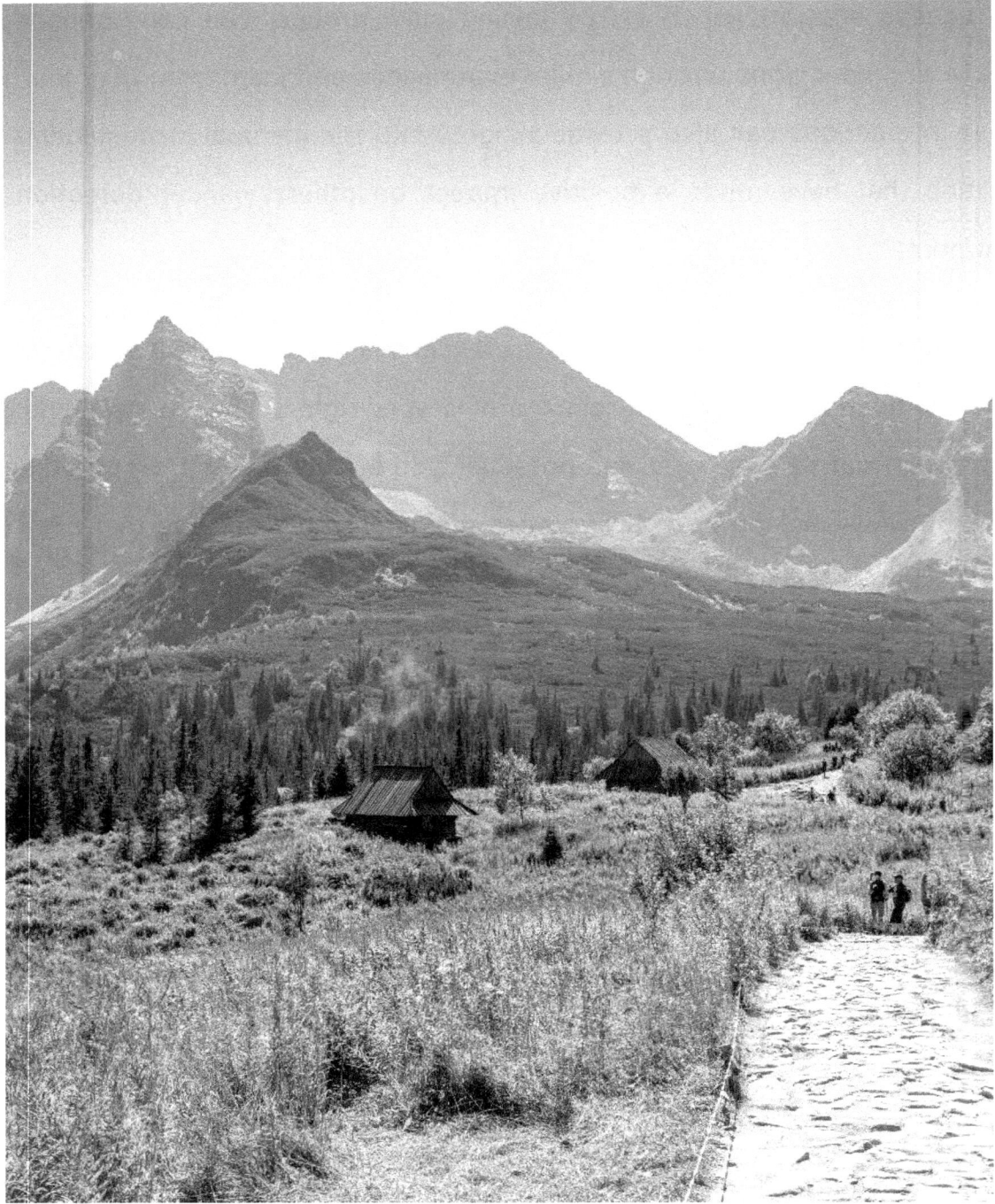

Chapter 8

Overcoming Barriers to Early Detection

Financial and Insurance Challenges

When it comes to cancer, the journey is not just physically and emotionally draining, but it can also take a toll on your finances. Dealing with the financial and insurance challenges that accompany a cancer diagnosis can be overwhelming, but it is essential to address them early on to ensure that you receive the best possible care without compromising your financial stability.

One of the first challenges you may encounter is the cost of cancer treatment. Cancer treatment can be expensive, and without proper insurance coverage, it may become a burden on your finances. It is crucial to understand your insurance policy thoroughly and be aware of what it covers. Review your policy, paying close attention to the deductible, co-pays, and out-of-pocket maximums. Consider seeking guidance from a financial advisor or reaching out to your insurance provider to clarify any uncertainties.

In some cases, even with insurance, the out-of-pocket expenses can be significant. This is where financial planning becomes crucial. Create a budget that accounts for medical expenses, medications, transportation costs, and potential loss of income due to treatment or recovery. Explore resources such as cancer-specific financial assistance programs, grants, or non-profit organizations that provide financial aid to cancer patients.

Another challenge you may face is navigating the complexities of health insurance. Understanding the terminology, coverage limitations, and pre-authorization requirements can be overwhelming. If you find yourself struggling, don't hesitate to reach out to a patient advocate or a social worker who can guide you through the process and help you make informed decisions. Additionally, consider keeping detailed records of all medical expenses, including bills, receipts, and insurance statements. This will prove invaluable when it comes to filing insurance claims or applying for financial assistance.

Furthermore, it is crucial to be proactive and take steps to protect your financial future. Consider exploring options such as disability insurance, critical illness insurance, or cancer-specific insurance policies that can provide additional coverage and financial support during your cancer journey.

While the financial and insurance challenges may seem daunting, it is important to remember that you are not alone. There are resources, organizations, and professionals dedicated to helping individuals navigate these challenges. By staying informed, seeking assistance when needed, and being proactive in your financial planning, you can alleviate some of the stress and focus on what truly matters – your health and well-being.

Cultural and Language Barriers

In the fight against cancer, it is crucial to recognize and address the various barriers that may hinder early detection and treatment. One significant obstacle that many individuals face is the presence of cultural and language barriers. Understanding and overcoming these barriers is essential to empower individuals from all backgrounds to detect cancer signs sooner and take prompt action.

Cultural diversity is a beautiful aspect of our society, but it can also present challenges when it comes to healthcare. Different cultures may have varying beliefs, attitudes, and practices regarding cancer. These cultural differences can influence how individuals perceive the disease, their willingness to seek medical help, and their adherence to treatment plans.

Language barriers further complicate matters, as effective communication is vital in conveying essential information about cancer awareness and prevention. Limited English proficiency can hinder access to healthcare services, understanding medical instructions, and participating in informed decision-making.

To bridge these gaps, it is crucial to promote cultural competence in healthcare by training healthcare professionals to understand and respect diverse cultural beliefs. By doing so, they can effectively communicate with patients and provide culturally sensitive care. Additionally, healthcare providers should strive to offer interpreter services or multilingual materials to ensure that language does not prevent individuals from receiving the care they need.

Education also plays a vital role in overcoming cultural and language barriers. By raising awareness about the importance of early cancer detection and debunking common misconceptions, we can empower individuals from all backgrounds to overcome cultural stigmas and seek timely medical help. This can be achieved through community outreach programs, informative workshops, and the dissemination of culturally appropriate educational materials.

Furthermore, collaborating with community leaders, cultural organizations, and religious institutions can help bridge the gap between healthcare providers and diverse communities. By fostering partnerships, we can better understand and address the unique challenges faced by different cultural groups, tailor educational materials to their specific needs, and facilitate access to cancer screening and treatment services.

In conclusion, cultural and language barriers pose significant challenges in the fight against cancer. However, by promoting cultural competence, providing language support, and educating communities, we can empower individuals from all backgrounds to recognize cancer signs sooner and take proactive steps towards early detection and treatment. Together, we can ensure that nobody is left behind in the battle against cancer.

Addressing Fear and Stigma

Fear and stigma surrounding cancer have long been significant barriers to early detection and treatment. In this subchapter, we will delve into the importance of addressing these emotions and misconceptions, providing valuable insights and strategies for overcoming them. By empowering individuals to confront their fears and dispel stigmas associated with cancer, we can create a more supportive and proactive approach to detecting signs and symptoms sooner.

Fear is a natural response when faced with the possibility of cancer. The uncertainty, potential pain, and life-altering consequences can be overwhelming. However, it is crucial to acknowledge and address these fears head-on. By doing so, individuals can take proactive steps towards detection, early intervention, and improved outcomes. This subchapter will explore various techniques to manage fear, including mindfulness exercises, seeking support from loved ones or support groups, and engaging in open conversations with healthcare professionals.

Stigma is another significant hurdle that must be confronted. The negative perceptions and stereotypes associated with cancer often lead to isolation, shame, and delayed diagnosis. By challenging misconceptions and promoting understanding, we can create a more inclusive and empathetic society. This subchapter will provide insights into debunking common myths surrounding cancer, encouraging open dialogue, and promoting education and awareness. Additionally, we will highlight the importance of destigmatizing cancer survivors and celebrating their resilience and strength.

To address fears and stigma effectively, it is essential to engage with diverse audiences. This book is aimed at everybody, regardless of their background or prior knowledge of cancer. By providing accessible information and relatable stories, we hope to empower individuals to recognize signs and symptoms sooner. Offering practical tips on self-examination, recognizing red flags, and seeking timely medical attention, this subchapter will equip readers with the necessary tools to take control of their health and well-being.

Ultimately, addressing fear and stigma surrounding cancer is a collective effort. It requires a shift in societal attitudes, increased awareness, and a supportive network of individuals who are willing to challenge misconceptions and provide emotional support. By fostering a culture that encourages open dialogue, empathy, and early detection, we can significantly improve outcomes for those affected by cancer.

In conclusion, this subchapter aims to empower individuals to confront and overcome their fears while dispelling stigmas associated with cancer. By providing valuable insights, strategies, and practical tips, we hope to create a more proactive and supportive society that works together to detect signs and symptoms sooner.

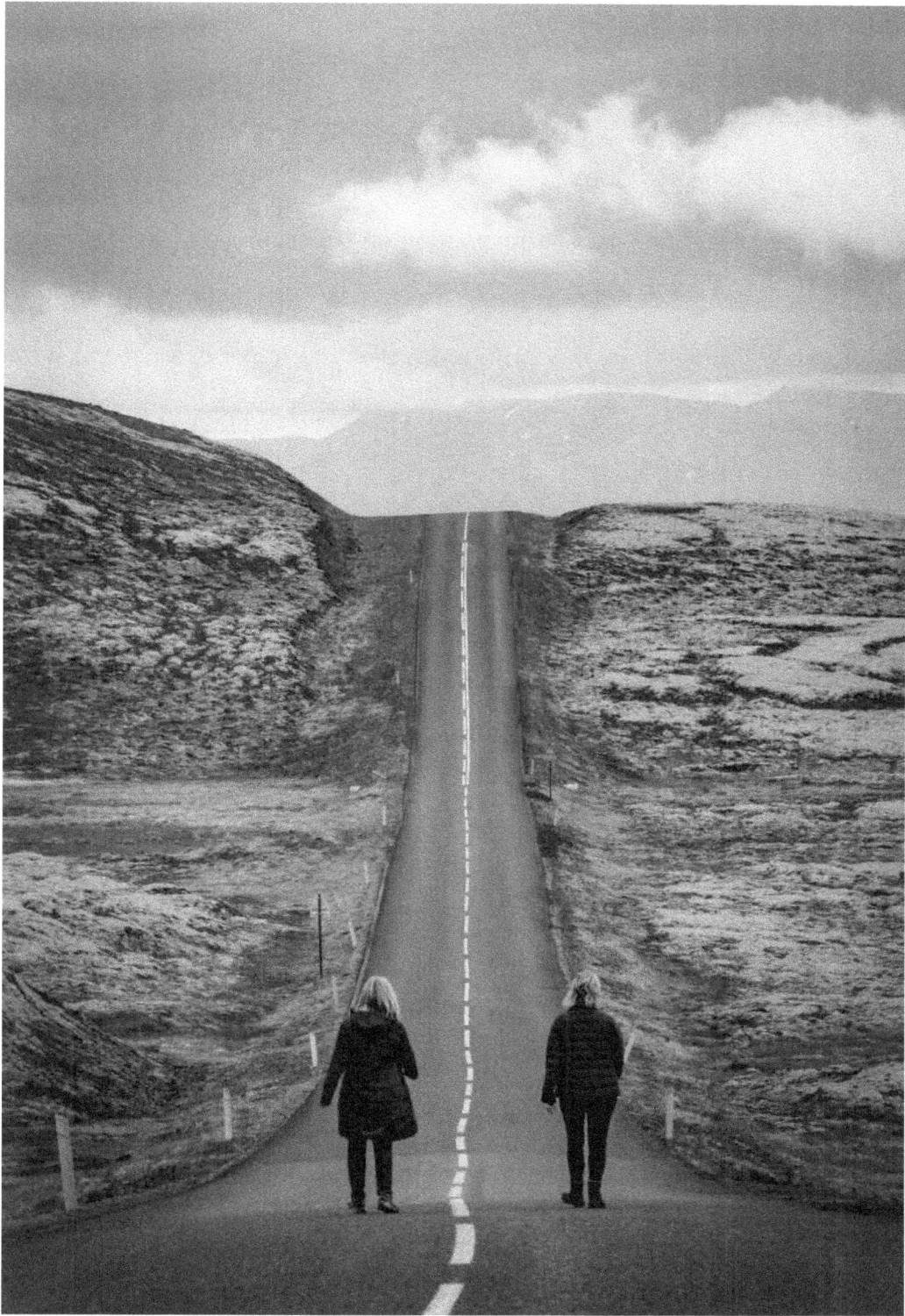

Chapter 9

Promoting Cancer Awareness in Communities

Community Outreach Programs

Community outreach programs play a crucial role in raising cancer awareness and empowering individuals to detect signs sooner. In this subchapter, we will delve into the significance of these programs and explore the various initiatives that exist to educate and support individuals in recognizing the signs and symptoms of cancer earlier.

Cancer awareness is essential for everyone, regardless of age, gender, or background. By creating community outreach programs, we can ensure that information about cancer detection and prevention reaches every corner of society. These programs aim to bridge the gap between medical professionals and the general public, providing accessible resources and knowledge to empower individuals in taking proactive steps towards their health.

One of the primary objectives of community outreach programs is education. By organizing workshops, seminars, and informational sessions, these programs equip individuals with the necessary knowledge to recognize the early signs of cancer. Educating the public about the common symptoms, risk factors, and available screening methods is crucial in enabling early detection, which significantly improves the chances of successful treatment.

Furthermore, community outreach programs often collaborate with healthcare professionals, local organizations, and volunteers to provide free or affordable cancer screenings. These screenings play a vital role in identifying potential cancer cases at an early stage, allowing for timely intervention and treatment. Additionally, these programs may also offer counseling services and support groups for individuals and families affected by cancer, fostering a sense of community and empowerment.

To ensure the effectiveness of community outreach programs, it is crucial to tailor them to the specific needs and demographics of the target audience. This means understanding the unique challenges faced by different communities and designing initiatives that are culturally sensitive and easily accessible. By engaging with various niches, such as "How to Discover Cancer Earlier: A Proactive Guide to Recognizing Signs and Symptoms Sooner," community outreach programs can address the specific concerns and misconceptions that may exist within different groups.

In conclusion, community outreach programs are powerful tools in raising cancer awareness and empowering individuals to detect signs sooner. By providing education, screenings, and support, these programs enable proactive action and improve the chances of successful treatment. It is essential for everyone to engage with these initiatives and spread the knowledge within their communities to ensure that no one is left behind in the fight against cancer. Together, we can create a society that is well-informed, proactive, and empowered in the face of this disease.

Collaboration with Local Organizations

In the fight against cancer, collaboration is key. No single entity can tackle this pervasive disease alone. This chapter explores the valuable role of collaboration with local organizations in raising cancer awareness and empowering individuals to detect signs sooner.

Local organizations play a vital role in cancer awareness as they possess an in-depth understanding of their communities. These organizations, ranging from community health centers to non-profit groups, are well-positioned to reach and engage diverse populations. By partnering with them, we can tap into their local knowledge, networks, and resources to create a more comprehensive and effective cancer awareness campaign.

One of the primary benefits of collaborating with local organizations is the ability to tailor our message to specific audiences. Cancer affects people from all walks of life, and different populations may have unique barriers to awareness and prevention. By working closely with local organizations, we can ensure that our message is culturally sensitive, linguistically appropriate, and resonates with the target audience.

Collaboration also enables us to leverage existing programs and initiatives. Local organizations often have ongoing projects related to health education and prevention. By joining forces, we can integrate cancer awareness into these existing efforts, maximizing resources and expanding our reach. For example, partnering with a local school district can help us incorporate cancer education into the curriculum, reaching not only students but also their families and the broader community.

Furthermore, collaboration fosters a sense of shared responsibility and collective action. By involving local organizations, we can create a network of stakeholders dedicated to promoting cancer awareness. This network can pool their expertise, efforts, and resources to achieve a common goal: empowering individuals to detect signs sooner. Together, we can organize community events, distribute educational materials, offer free screenings, and provide support services to those affected by cancer.

In conclusion, collaboration with local organizations is a vital component of our cancer awareness campaign. By partnering with these organizations, we can tap into their local knowledge, tailor our message to specific populations, leverage existing programs, and foster a sense of shared responsibility. Together, we can empower individuals to detect signs of cancer sooner and make a meaningful impact on the fight against this disease.

Advocacy and Policy Initiatives

In the fight against cancer, advocacy and policy initiatives play a crucial role in raising awareness, promoting early detection, and improving the overall well-being of individuals affected by this devastating disease. This chapter will delve into the significance of advocacy and policy initiatives in the realm of cancer awareness and prevention, highlighting their impact on empowering individuals to detect signs sooner.

Advocacy serves as a powerful tool to bring attention to cancer-related issues and to advocate for policy changes that can save lives. It involves individuals, organizations, and communities coming together to raise their voices, share personal experiences, and push for positive change. By spreading awareness about the importance of early detection and the availability of screening programs, advocacy efforts aim to empower individuals to take charge of their health and make informed decisions.

Policy initiatives, on the other hand, focus on implementing systemic changes at a governmental level to improve cancer detection, prevention, and treatment. These initiatives can encompass a wide range of measures, including the development of public health campaigns, the establishment of screening guidelines, the provision of funding for research and treatment, and the enforcement of regulations to reduce exposure to carcinogens.

By combining advocacy and policy initiatives, we can create an environment that supports early detection and prevention. Through public health campaigns and educational programs, individuals can learn about the signs and symptoms of cancer, understand the importance of regular screenings, and gain knowledge about risk factors and preventive measures. These initiatives also aim to eliminate barriers to access to healthcare services, ensuring that everyone, regardless of their socioeconomic status, has the opportunity to detect cancer early and receive timely treatment.

Furthermore, advocacy and policy initiatives seek to promote research and innovation in the field of cancer detection. By supporting funding for research institutions and encouraging collaboration between scientists and medical professionals, we can advance the development of new diagnostic tools and screening techniques, ultimately leading to earlier detection and improved survival rates.

In conclusion, advocacy and policy initiatives are vital components in the comprehensive approach to cancer awareness. By raising awareness, promoting early detection, and advocating for policy changes, we can empower individuals to detect signs sooner, ultimately saving lives and improving the well-being of individuals and communities affected by cancer. Together, we can make a difference and create a future where cancer is detected earlier, treated effectively, and, ultimately, prevented.

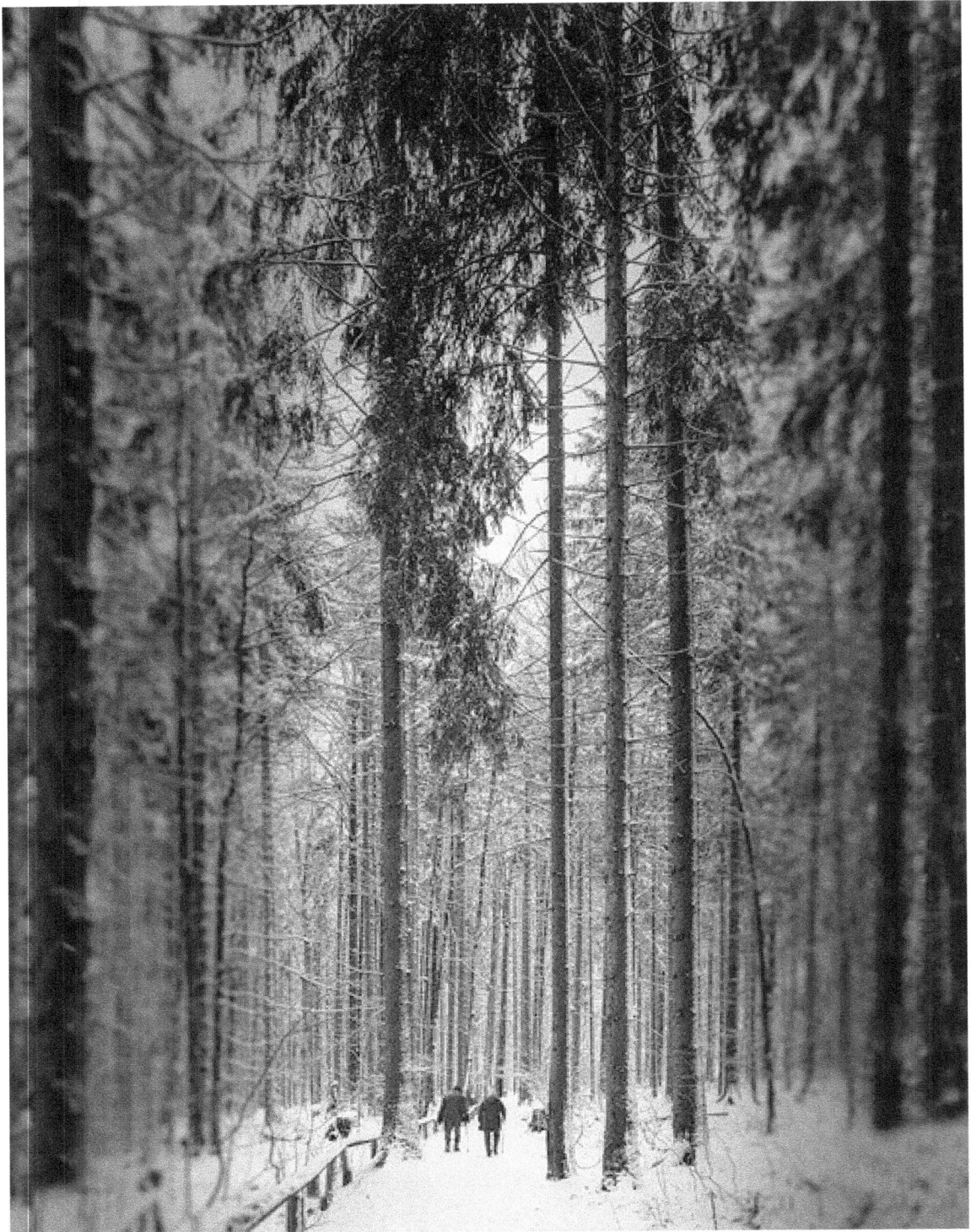

Chapter 10

Inspiring Stories of Early Detection

Real-life Experiences of Early Diagnosis

In this subchapter, we delve into the real-life experiences of individuals who have been diagnosed with cancer at an early stage. These stories serve as powerful examples of the impact early detection can have on the outcome of the disease. By sharing their journeys, we hope to inspire and empower readers to take charge of their health and recognize the signs and symptoms of cancer sooner.

Meet Sarah, a vibrant and energetic woman in her early thirties. During a routine check-up, her doctor discovered a lump in her breast. Sarah, being proactive about her health, immediately sought further investigation. The early diagnosis allowed her to undergo treatment promptly, resulting in successful removal of the cancer and a full recovery. Sarah's story highlights the importance of self-examination and regular check-ups, regardless of age or perceived risk.

Next, we meet John, a middle-aged man who experienced persistent fatigue and unexplained weight loss. Concerned about his symptoms, he visited his doctor and insisted on further tests. The diagnosis revealed cancer in its early stages, which was successfully treated. John's proactive approach saved his life, emphasizing the significance of recognizing and acting upon unusual changes in the body.

In another story, we encounter Susan, a young mother who noticed abnormal bleeding between menstrual cycles. Despite being busy with her family responsibilities, Susan prioritized her health and sought medical attention. The early diagnosis of cervical cancer allowed for less invasive treatment, preserving her fertility and enabling her to continue being there for her children. Susan's experience demonstrates the importance of listening to your body and seeking medical advice when something feels off.

These real-life experiences illustrate that cancer does not discriminate based on age, gender, or lifestyle. Early detection is crucial for everyone, and these individuals' stories highlight the potential positive outcomes of proactive health management. By being vigilant and aware of changes in our bodies, we can increase the chances of catching cancer in its early stages when treatment options are more effective.

Whether you are a young adult, a middle-aged individual, or a senior citizen, recognizing the signs and symptoms of cancer earlier can be a game-changer. This subchapter serves as a reminder that we all have the power to take control of our health and detect cancer sooner. By learning from these real-life experiences, we can empower ourselves and others to become proactive in the fight against cancer. Remember, knowledge is key, and early detection can save lives.

Personal Testimonies and Lessons Learned

In this subchapter, we delve into the powerful stories of individuals who have battled cancer and the valuable lessons they have learned along the way. By sharing these personal testimonies and experiences, we hope to inspire and educate readers about the importance of early detection and recognizing the signs and symptoms of cancer sooner.

1. Jane's Story: A Journey of Strength and Resilience

Jane, a vibrant and active woman in her forties, discovered a lump in her breast during a routine self-examination. Despite her initial fear, she promptly sought medical attention and was diagnosed with breast cancer in its early stages. Through her journey, Jane realized the significance of actively examining her body and being aware of any changes. Her story serves as a reminder that early detection can significantly increase the chances of successful treatment.

2. Mark's Testimony: The Importance of Regular Screenings

Mark, a middle-aged man, had always been diligent about his health. However, it was during a routine colonoscopy that doctors discovered a precancerous polyp. Mark's experience highlights the vital role that regular screenings play in detecting cancer at its earliest stages, even when no symptoms are present. His story emphasizes the importance of scheduling recommended screenings and being proactive about one's health.

3. Sarah's Journey: A Lesson in Listening to Your Body

Sarah, a busy working mother, ignored persistent stomach pain for months until it became unbearable. After finally seeking medical help, she was diagnosed with ovarian cancer, already in an advanced stage. Sarah's experience teaches us the importance of listening to our bodies and seeking medical attention when something doesn't feel right. She encourages readers not to dismiss subtle symptoms and to trust their instincts.

These personal testimonies highlight the diverse range of experiences individuals have faced when confronted with cancer. They serve as a reminder that cancer can affect anyone, regardless of age, gender, or lifestyle. By sharing these stories, "Cancer Awareness for All" aims to empower readers to take charge of their health, be vigilant in monitoring their bodies, and seek medical attention promptly when needed.

Through these narratives, readers will gain insights into the journeys of these courageous individuals, understanding the importance of early detection and the impact it can have on treatment outcomes. The lessons learned from these experiences will inspire readers to become proactive in recognizing the signs and symptoms of cancer earlier, ultimately leading to better outcomes and improved survival rates. With knowledge and awareness, we can all contribute to the fight against cancer and empower ourselves and our loved ones to live healthier lives.

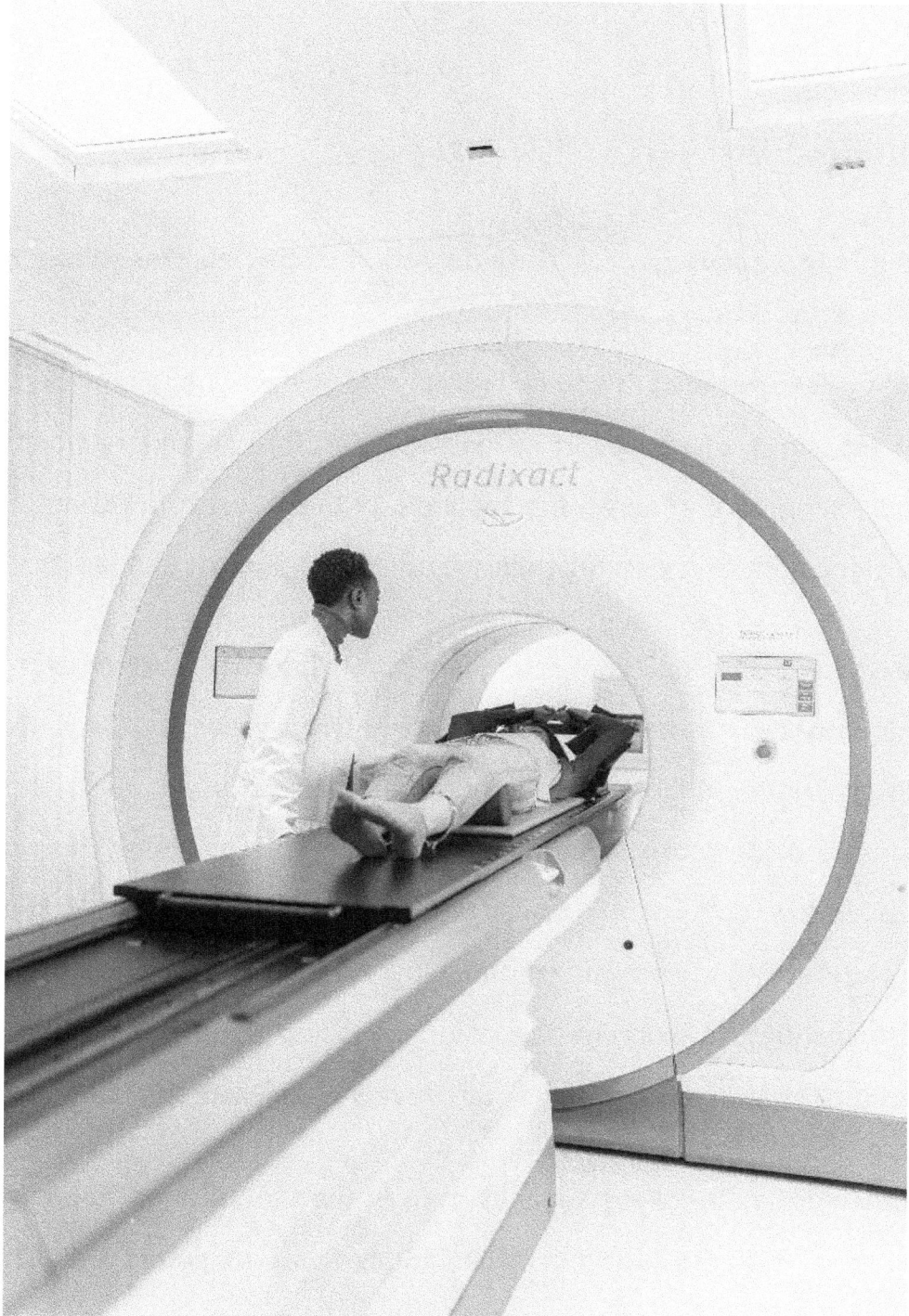

Chapter 11

The Future of Cancer Detection

Advancements in Screening Technology

In the fight against cancer, early detection is crucial. The sooner cancer is detected, the better the chances of successful treatment and a positive outcome. Fortunately, advancements in screening technology have made it easier than ever to detect the signs of cancer at an early stage. This subchapter explores the various advancements in screening technology that are empowering individuals to detect signs sooner and take proactive measures against cancer.

One of the most significant advancements in cancer screening technology is the development of more accurate and efficient screening tests. Traditional screening methods, such as mammograms and colonoscopies, have been improved to provide more reliable results. For example, digital mammography allows for clearer and more detailed images of breast tissue, increasing the chances of detecting abnormalities. Similarly, virtual colonoscopy uses advanced imaging techniques to examine the colon, reducing the discomfort associated with traditional colonoscopies while still providing accurate results.

Another groundbreaking advancement is the rise of liquid biopsies. These tests analyze a patient's blood or other bodily fluids to detect the presence of cancer cells or genetic mutations associated with cancer. Liquid biopsies offer a less invasive alternative to traditional tissue biopsies, allowing for earlier and more frequent testing. They are particularly useful in monitoring cancer patients for recurrence and tracking treatment effectiveness.

Furthermore, advancements in imaging technology have revolutionized cancer screening. Techniques such as positron emission tomography (PET) and magnetic resonance imaging (MRI) provide detailed images of the body, helping to identify tumors and determine their stage. These imaging techniques are non-invasive and can detect cancer in its early stages, allowing for prompt treatment.

Moreover, the advent of artificial intelligence (AI) has significantly improved cancer screening and diagnosis. AI algorithms can analyze vast amounts of data, including medical images and patient records, to identify patterns and potential indicators of cancer. This technology helps doctors make more accurate diagnoses and develop personalized treatment plans tailored to each patient's unique circumstances.

In conclusion, advancements in screening technology have revolutionized cancer detection and empowered individuals to detect signs of the disease sooner. From more accurate and efficient screening tests to liquid biopsies, imaging technology, and AI, the tools available to detect cancer early have never been more advanced. By staying informed about these advancements and taking advantage of the latest screening technologies, individuals can play an active role in their own cancer awareness and take proactive steps towards early detection and successful treatment.

Promising Research and Innovations

In recent years, the field of cancer research has witnessed incredible advancements and breakthroughs, offering hope to millions of individuals affected by this devastating disease. From improved diagnostic tools to cutting-edge treatments, innovative research has paved the way for earlier detection and more effective interventions in the fight against cancer.

One of the most promising areas of research lies in the development of advanced screening techniques. Traditional cancer screening methods, such as mammograms and colonoscopies, have proven to be valuable tools in detecting cancer at earlier stages. However, they are not foolproof and often miss certain types of cancers. Researchers are now exploring alternative methods, such as liquid biopsies and molecular profiling, which can provide a more comprehensive and accurate assessment of an individual's cancer risk.

Liquid biopsies, for instance, involve analyzing a patient's blood sample to identify genetic mutations or tumor-derived materials. This non-invasive method has shown great potential in detecting cancer at its earliest stages, even before symptoms manifest. Similarly, molecular profiling utilizes advanced genomic technology to analyze the genetic makeup of tumors, allowing for personalized treatment plans tailored to each patient's specific cancer profile.

Another groundbreaking innovation in cancer research is immunotherapy. This revolutionary approach harnesses the body's immune system to target and destroy cancer cells. By boosting the immune response, immunotherapy has shown remarkable success in treating various types of cancer, including lung, melanoma, and leukemia. Researchers continue to explore different immunotherapeutic strategies, such as checkpoint inhibitors and CAR-T cell therapy, to further enhance treatment outcomes and extend the benefits to a wider range of cancer patients.

Moreover, the field of precision medicine holds tremendous promise in the fight against cancer. This approach involves analyzing a patient's unique genetic and molecular characteristics to develop personalized treatment plans. By tailoring therapies to an individual's specific needs, precision medicine aims to maximize treatment effectiveness while minimizing side effects. This transformative concept has the potential to revolutionize cancer care, offering patients more targeted and efficient treatments.

As we delve into the world of cancer research and innovation, it becomes evident that the future holds great promise for early detection and effective treatment. These advancements not only empower individuals to take charge of their health but also provide hope for a world where cancer is no longer a life-threatening disease. By staying informed and supporting ongoing research efforts, we can all contribute to the collective fight against cancer and create a brighter future for everyone.

Hope and Optimism for Early Detection

In the fight against cancer, hope and optimism play a crucial role in empowering individuals to detect signs sooner. This subchapter aims to instill a sense of positivity and motivation in every reader, regardless of their background or current knowledge about cancer. By highlighting the importance of early detection and the potential for positive outcomes, we hope to encourage a proactive mindset in the face of this formidable disease.

Cancer is a word that strikes fear into the hearts of many, but it is important to remember that early detection can significantly improve survival rates. By understanding the signs and symptoms of various types of cancer, we can equip ourselves with the tools necessary to detect it sooner. This knowledge empowers us to take control of our health and seek medical attention promptly, increasing the chances of successful treatment and recovery.

It is natural to feel overwhelmed when faced with the possibility of cancer, but it is essential to focus on the positive aspects of early detection. By catching cancer in its early stages, treatment options are often less invasive and more effective. This can lead to a better quality of life during and after treatment, providing hope for a brighter future.

Moreover, advancements in medical technology and research have paved the way for early detection methods that were once unimaginable. From innovative screening techniques to genetic testing, the possibilities for identifying cancer at its earliest and most treatable stages are constantly expanding. By staying informed and proactive, we can make use of these tools and increase our chances of detecting cancer before it spreads.

This subchapter will provide valuable insights into the proactive steps we can take to recognize signs and symptoms of cancer sooner. From understanding our body's warning signals to adopting healthy lifestyle habits, each individual can play an active role in their own health. By embracing hope and optimism, we can overcome any fears or uncertainties and embark on a journey of early detection and prevention.

Let us come together as a community and empower one another to be vigilant about cancer awareness. By sharing stories of survival and encouragement, we can create a support network that fosters hope and optimism. Together, we can raise awareness, break down barriers, and ensure that nobody faces cancer alone.

Whether you are a cancer survivor, a caregiver, or simply someone who wants to be proactive about their health, this subchapter is for you. Let us embark on this journey of hope and optimism, knowing that early detection holds the key to a brighter future. Together, we can make a difference and empower individuals to detect signs of cancer sooner.

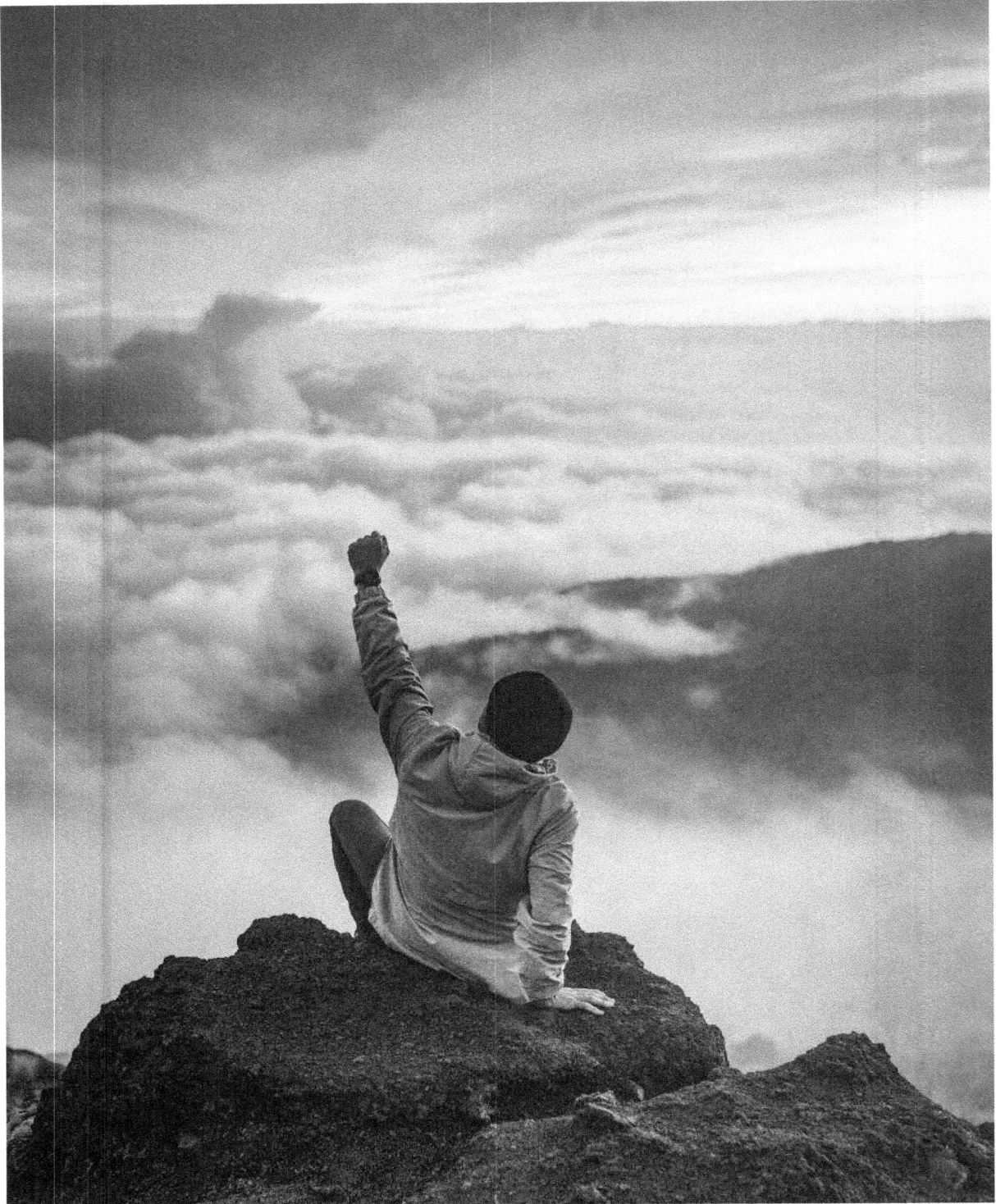

Chapter 12

Taking Action: Spreading Cancer Awareness

Becoming an Advocate in Your Community

In the fight against cancer, every individual has the power to make a difference. By becoming an advocate in your community, you can play a vital role in raising awareness, promoting early detection, and supporting those affected by this devastating disease. "Cancer Awareness for All: Empowering Individuals to Detect Signs Sooner" is a comprehensive guide that equips everybody with the knowledge and tools to become an effective advocate.

Advocacy starts with education. By educating yourself and staying informed about various types of cancers, their signs, symptoms, and risk factors, you can empower yourself to recognize warning signs earlier. This book, "How to Discover Cancer Earlier: A Proactive Guide to Recognizing Signs and Symptoms Sooner," serves as a valuable resource to help you understand the importance of early detection and equip you with the necessary information to identify potential signs of cancer.

Once you have gained knowledge about cancer, it's time to spread awareness in your community. Organize and participate in events such as cancer awareness walks, health fairs, and fundraising campaigns. Use social media platforms to share educational content, personal stories, and resources that can help individuals take proactive steps towards early detection. By engaging with your community, you can encourage people to prioritize their health and seek medical attention if they notice any concerning symptoms.

Supporting those affected by cancer is another crucial aspect of advocacy. Reach out to local cancer support groups, hospitals, and nonprofits to find ways to offer assistance. Volunteer your time, donate resources, or provide emotional support to cancer patients, survivors, and their families. By lending a helping hand, you can make a significant impact in their lives and provide them with the strength and encouragement they need during their journey.

Remember, advocacy is not limited to individuals directly affected by cancer. It is a responsibility that falls upon all of us. By becoming an advocate in your community, you can help save lives by promoting early detection, supporting those affected by cancer, and spreading awareness about the importance of proactive healthcare practices. "Cancer Awareness for All: Empowering Individuals to Detect Signs Sooner" is your guide to understanding and fulfilling this crucial role. Together, we can make a difference and empower individuals to detect signs of cancer sooner.

Promoting Cancer Awareness on Social Media

In today's digital age, social media has become a powerful tool for spreading information and raising awareness on various topics. When it comes to cancer, harnessing the potential of these platforms can make a significant difference in early detection and prevention. This subchapter explores the importance of promoting cancer awareness on social media and how it can empower individuals to detect signs sooner.

Social media platforms offer an unprecedented reach to a diverse audience, making them ideal for disseminating vital information about cancer. By leveraging these platforms, we can engage everybody, regardless of age, gender, or background, in the conversation about cancer awareness. Through captivating content, informative posts, and engaging campaigns, we can educate individuals about the importance of early detection and equip them with the knowledge to recognize potential signs and symptoms.

One of the key advantages of utilizing social media is its ability to transcend geographical boundaries. Cancer affects people globally, and by utilizing social media, we can create a global network of support and awareness. By connecting individuals from different walks of life, we can foster a sense of community and encourage open conversations about cancer detection. Sharing personal stories, experiences, and testimonials can help break down stigma and motivate others to seek medical advice when necessary.

Moreover, social media provides an ideal platform for sharing infographics, videos, and interactive content that simplifies complex medical information. By presenting information in a visually appealing and easily consumable format, we can capture the attention of a wider audience, including those who may not actively seek out cancer-related information. Through engaging campaigns, challenges, and hashtags, we can encourage individuals to participate actively, spreading awareness to their own networks and amplifying the message.

In order to promote cancer awareness effectively on social media, collaboration with influencers, healthcare professionals, and cancer survivors is crucial. By partnering with influential individuals who have a large following, we can leverage their platforms to reach a broader audience. Similarly, involving healthcare professionals and cancer survivors in awareness campaigns can add credibility and provide valuable insights into the detection and treatment process.

In conclusion, social media platforms offer an incredible opportunity to promote cancer awareness to everybody. By harnessing the power of these platforms, we can engage a diverse audience, break down barriers, and empower individuals to detect signs and symptoms of cancer sooner. Through informative content, interactive campaigns, and collaboration with influencers, we can create a global network of support and awareness, ultimately saving lives through early detection and prevention.

Organizing Fundraisers and Events

Fundraisers and events play a crucial role in raising awareness about cancer and supporting those affected by the disease. By organizing and participating in such activities, we can make a significant impact on the lives of individuals and their families. This subchapter provides practical guidance on how to plan and execute successful fundraisers and events, enabling everyone to contribute to the cause of cancer awareness.

1. Setting the Purpose:
Before organizing any fundraiser or event, it is essential to define the purpose clearly. Are you raising funds for research, supporting cancer patients, or spreading awareness? Identifying the goal will help you structure your event effectively.

2. Brainstorming Ideas:

Consider various event ideas that align with your purpose. Some popular options include charity walks, benefit concerts, auctions, and community fairs. Think about what suits your target audience and the resources available to you.

3. Assembling a Team:

Form a passionate and dedicated team to help you plan and execute the event. Delegate responsibilities and ensure everyone is committed to the cause. Remember, teamwork is key to the success of any fundraiser or event.

4. Securing Sponsorships:

Reach out to local businesses, organizations, and individuals who may be interested in sponsoring your event. Offer them different sponsorship packages in exchange for their support. Sponsors can contribute funds, resources, or even provide venues for your event.

5. Spreading the Word:

Create a comprehensive marketing plan to generate awareness about your fundraiser or event. Utilize social media platforms, local newspapers, radio stations, and community bulletin boards to reach a broader audience. Personal connections and word-of-mouth promotion can also be incredibly effective.

6. Logistics and Execution:

Pay attention to the smallest details, such as permits, insurance, security, and parking arrangements. Plan your event schedule, including registration, speakers, entertainment, and any other activities. Ensure everything runs smoothly on the day of the event.

7. Engaging Participants:

Provide opportunities for participants to engage and contribute. Offer merchandise, food stalls, or educational booths where attendees can learn more about cancer prevention and early detection. Remember to express gratitude to all participants and volunteers for their support.

By organizing fundraisers and events, we can create a united front against cancer, encouraging earlier detection and improving the lives of those affected by the disease. Whether you choose to host a small gathering or a large-scale event, every effort counts. Together, let's empower individuals to recognize the signs and symptoms of cancer sooner and work towards a world where cancer is detected early, treated effectively, and prevented altogether.

Conclusion

Empowering Everyone to Detect Cancer Signs Sooner

Recap of Key Takeaways

Throughout this book, we have explored the crucial topic of early cancer detection and the importance of recognizing signs and symptoms sooner. By empowering ourselves with knowledge, we can play an active role in our own health and potentially save lives.

Here are some key takeaways to remember:

1. Importance of Awareness: Cancer is a prevalent disease that affects millions of lives worldwide. By raising our awareness about the signs and symptoms, we can detect cancer at an earlier stage, increasing the chances of successful treatment and recovery.

2. Knowing the Red Flags: Familiarize yourself with the common warning signs of cancer, such as unexplained weight loss, persistent fatigue, changes in bowel or bladder habits, and unusual lumps or growths. Recognizing these indicators can prompt timely medical attention.

3. Regular Check-ups and Screenings: Establish a routine of regular health check-ups and cancer screenings. Early detection often relies on these proactive measures, especially for common cancers like breast, cervical, colon, and prostate.

4. Self-Examination: Learn how to perform self-examinations, such as breast self-exams or skin checks, to spot any abnormalities. Remember, early detection starts with knowing your body and being attentive to changes.

5. Lifestyle Modifications: Adopting a healthy lifestyle can reduce your risk of developing cancer. Incorporate regular exercise, a balanced diet, limited alcohol consumption, and no smoking into your daily routine.

6. Educate Others: Share your knowledge with family, friends, and colleagues. By spreading awareness, you can help others recognize signs and symptoms earlier, potentially saving lives.

7. Trusting Medical Professionals: If you notice any concerning signs, don't hesitate to consult with a healthcare professional. They are equipped to assess your symptoms, perform necessary tests, and provide appropriate guidance.

Remember, cancer awareness is not limited to a particular age group or gender. It is relevant to everybody, as early detection can make a significant difference in treatment outcomes. By embracing a proactive approach and staying informed, we can empower ourselves to detect cancer signs sooner, potentially saving lives and fostering a healthier future for all.

Take charge of your health today and join the movement towards empowering individuals to detect cancer earlier. Together, we can make a difference!

ENCOURAGEMENT FOR PROACTIVE STEPS

In the fight against cancer, proactive steps play a crucial role in detecting signs and symptoms earlier, ultimately leading to better treatment outcomes. This subchapter aims to inspire and empower individuals from all walks of life to take charge of their health and become active participants in the battle against cancer.

Cancer Awareness for All: Empowering Individuals to Detect Signs Sooner is a book dedicated to spreading knowledge and awareness about this devastating disease. Its goal is to equip everybody, regardless of their background or medical expertise, with the tools they need to recognize the early warning signs of cancer.

Taking proactive steps involves a combination of education, self-awareness, and regular health check-ups. It begins with understanding your own body and being attuned to any changes that may occur. By familiarizing yourself with the common signs and symptoms of different types of cancer, you can become an active participant in your own healthcare.

The importance of regular check-ups cannot be stressed enough. Scheduling routine screenings and examinations can help detect cancer in its early stages, when it is most treatable. By prioritizing your health and making these appointments a part of your regular healthcare routine, you are taking a significant step towards early detection.

Furthermore, this subchapter emphasizes the role of self-advocacy in the fight against cancer. It encourages individuals to become their own health advocates, asking questions, seeking second opinions, and staying informed about the latest advancements in cancer research and treatment. By actively participating in your own healthcare decisions, you can ensure that your concerns are addressed and your needs are met.

Lastly, this subchapter highlights the importance of emotional support and encouragement. A cancer diagnosis can be overwhelming, but having a strong support system can make all the difference. Friends, family, and support groups can provide comfort, guidance, and motivation throughout the cancer journey.

In conclusion, this subchapter serves as a reminder that each one of us has the power to make a difference in the fight against cancer. By taking proactive steps, educating ourselves, prioritizing our health, advocating for our well-being, and seeking support, we can empower ourselves and others to detect the signs of cancer sooner. Together, we can make a significant impact in the battle against this disease and improve the chances of successful treatment.

Final Thoughts on the Importance of Early Detection

In our journey through this book, "Cancer Awareness for All: Empowering Individuals to Detect Signs Sooner," we have delved deep into the crucial topic of early detection of cancer. We have explored various types of cancer, their signs and symptoms, and the proactive steps one can take to recognize them sooner. As we come to the end of this enlightening subchapter, let us reflect on the significance of early detection and its impact on our lives.

Cancer is a formidable opponent that affects millions of individuals worldwide. It does not discriminate based on age, gender, or lifestyle. Thus, it is essential for everybody to be aware of the signs and symptoms associated with different types of cancer. By understanding these warning signs, we can empower ourselves to take action and seek medical attention promptly.

Early detection plays a pivotal role in the successful treatment and management of cancer. The earlier cancer is detected, the greater the chances of a positive outcome. By recognizing the signs sooner, individuals can undergo necessary screenings, tests, and consultations with healthcare professionals. This proactive approach enables doctors to diagnose cancer at an early stage, when it is most treatable and before it spreads to other parts of the body.

Moreover, early detection not only improves the chances of survival but also reduces the need for aggressive and invasive treatment options. It allows for more conservative approaches, such as targeted therapies or minimally invasive surgeries, which often result in better quality of life for patients.

Early detection also offers the opportunity to educate ourselves and our loved ones about the preventive measures we can take to reduce the risk of developing cancer. By adopting a healthy lifestyle, including regular exercise, a balanced diet, and avoiding tobacco and excessive alcohol consumption, we can significantly reduce our chances of developing certain types of cancer.

In conclusion, the importance of early detection cannot be overstated. This subchapter has equipped us with the knowledge and tools necessary to recognize the signs and symptoms of cancer sooner. By being proactive and vigilant, we can empower ourselves to take control of our health and potentially save lives. Remember, early detection is the key to a brighter future, and together, we can make a difference in the fight against cancer.

AUTHOR NOTES & ACKNOWLEDGMENTS

First and foremost, I would like to express my deepest gratitude to the people who inspired and supported me throughout the journey of writing this book. This project would not have been possible without their unwavering belief in me and their invaluable contributions.

To my wife, thank you for your constant encouragement and understanding. Your love and support have been my anchor during the challenging times of researching and writing this book. Your belief in my ability to make a difference in people's lives has been my driving force.

I would also like to disclose that this book contains some renewed artificial intelligence-generated content. I really appreciate very recent technological innovation by outstanding scientists and of course our reader's understanding.

Lastly, I want to express my deepest gratitude to the readers of this book. I sincerely hope the strategies and methods outlined within these pages will provide you with the knowledge and tools needed to truly make your life much better. Your commitment to seeking any good solutions and willingness to explore multiple methods is commendable.

AUTHOR BIO

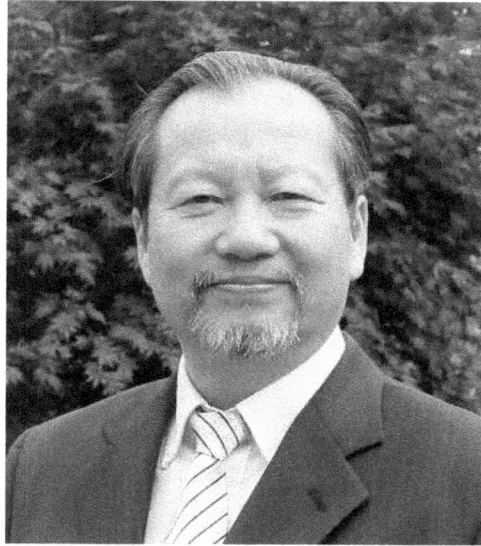

Johnson Wu earned his MD in 1982. With over 40 years of clinical experience, he has worked in hospitals in Zhejiang and Shanghai, China, as well as the Royal Marsden Hospital in London, UK.

On the recommendation of Sir Aaron Klug, the president of The Royal Society and a Nobel Prize winner in Chemistry, Dr. Wu was honorably awarded a British Royal Society Fellowship. He has published medical books and articles in seven countries and currently practices medicine in Toronto, Canada.